# THE MUSCLE FACTORY

## THE ULTIMATE GUIDE TO YOUR CUSTOM TRAINING PROGRAM FOR ACHIEVING THE LEAN, AESTHETIC BODY YOU'VE ALWAYS DREAMED OF

---

*A guide to create a basic, biological and scientific approach to building muscle and getting fit. Going deep into training and nutrition. Helping people get fit, fight against bro science and the no BS guide to supplements.*

By

*SCOTT OTERI*

Copyright © 2015

# TABLE OF CONTENTS

**Chapters**                                    **Contents**

## SECTION-I

### NUTRITION

## SECTION-II
## TRAINING

# What you will be able to achieve after reading this book

*No need to starve yourself or spend countless hours in the gym or a lot of money on useless pills and supplements. Get to the scientific basis of fitness training and figure out your own training and diet program.*

This book provides you a customized training program to achieve the aesthetic lean body, you have always wanted.  This book is a scientific and biological approach to fitness training.

- The best thing about this book is that it provides a custom crafted training program according to your body type. You can figure out your own diet plan and exercise program in accordance with your body type. So, after reading this book you will have a plan for yourself.

- Everything is logically proven and scientifically explained. So, you will have a deep insight of your training program after reading this book.

- A comprehensive diet chart is present in the "Nutrition" section, which describes the food sources recommended for every body type.

- Two Ultimate Programs for Beginners and Advanced Beginners are described to guide you through your training. Most common and effective exercises are explained step by step in the exercise catalog. The right way to do every exercise is explained.

- Be the master of your own body by controlling your mind and learn to develop the willpower, self-discipline and motivation it takes to build your ideal body.

- Interesting facts about the human body that you did not know before are scattered throughout the book.

- So, whether you are lean or obese, this book provides you a perfect and comprehensive pathway towards your ideal body, you always dreamt of.

# Disclaimer:

# About The Author

I'm Scott (I am Austro-American) and my mission is to help people achieve their dream bodies and health goals. It doesn't matter if you want to get lean, shredded or put that muscle mass on. I have the recipes you are searching for!

I love working as a fitness trainer and nutritional expert, and I have supported hundreds of clients with their health issues, physical and athletic goals! The natural next step for me was to write these simple steps down and provide workable, proven advice, grounded in science! I am not here to give you weird tips or sell supplements!

I myself was once confused about the basics of bodybuilding and was going nowhere but then I started taking the scientific approach and everything changed! I studied everything related to bodybuilding and metabolism of human body. I applied this knowledge on myself and the results were remarkable.
I want to spread the knowledge I have and when your body is transformed because of me, I will take pride in that. I want to share with you everything I know! I hope you enjoy my books and I would love to read your reviews on my tips.

I am Dr. Haroon Shabbir. I am a Medical Doctor specializing in Nutrition and Fitness. I helped Scott in completing this book. I added the scientific and medical basis to this book and explained everything with logic.

I am also the Consulting Physician at a Gym. I perform clinical and nutritional assessment of the clients and monitor their improvement.
I guide my patients towards a healthy nutrition and lifestyle. This book is a perfect way to spread the knowledge I have, to thousands of people.

We worked as a team and gathered all the knowledge we have and put it into this book. So, this book depicts the strength training from the viewpoint of both a Fitness Trainer and a Doctor.

# Chapter 1

## <u>What's your Body Type?</u>

The human body is divided into three main body types according to its shape, which are endomorph, ectomorph and mesomorph, (''-morph'' means shape). The body types are predetermined by your genes and cannot be changed.

**Ectomorphs** are the naturally lean and they seem to stay that way, despite eating a lot and spending a lot of time in the gym. They have a low body fat percentage and face difficulty in building muscle.

If you are an ectomorph, you should consume a good amount of calorie dense carbs and proteins, in order to build your muscle mass. You have to work hard to gain weight and you should NOT do too much cardio.

**Endomorphs** are the ones who are naturally overweight and are more at risk of getting obese. They usually have a high body fat percentage. They look pear-shaped as they have a high tendency to store body fat in abdomen.
If you are an endomorph, you should watch your carbohydrate intake and you should train with a higher intensity. You should eat non-calorie dense food. You are advised to do a lot of cardio.

**Mesomorphs** are the naturally muscular ones. They can increase their muscle mass easily. They usually have a normal fat percentage. Their body usually looks well-built and they have a high metabolic rate.
If you are a mesomorph, I have good news for you. You can have an ideal body easily without doing much of hard work. But do not take it lightly, you should train like an athlete and try to achieve higher goals.
In short, these are some fancy words for thin, heavy and muscular people respectively.

Experts say that you should train smart, not hard. So, you should know your body type to modify and focus your efforts and energy and maximize your potential to achieve a single 'goal', that is an ideal body.

# Chapter 2

## Analyzing your Body

This chapter includes, how to measure your body fat percentages, weight for height, muscle mass and BMI etc. Everyone should know these values for themselves and then try to move towards better numbers.

You should analyze these values periodically during your training. This will help you determine whether your body is making progress or not and how fast you are making progress.

### BODY FAT PERCENTAGE

This is a measure of total body fat in relation to the total body weight. People with fat percentages above 25% are considered as obese. On the other hand, a fat percentage less than 5 % is also considered unhealthy because a certain amount of fat is necessary for some body functions including hormone production and vitamin absorption.

Both, very high and very low body fat can be dangerous for the body. The body fat percentage is defined as total body fat, divided by total body mass. Normal percentages are given in the following table:

| Body Fat Percentage Chart | | |
|---|---|---|
| Description | Men | Women |
| Essential fat | 2-5% | 10-13% |
| Athletes | 6-13% | 14-20% |
| Fitness | 14-17% | 21-24% |
| Average | 18-24% | 25-31% |
| Obese | 25%+ | 32%+ |

It is a good parameter for getting an idea about your current status as well as calculating the progress of a person towards your ideal body.

## BMI

Body mass index or BMI is the most comprehensive parameter for indicating your overall health status. It is calculated by using the two variables of height and weight under the following formula:

$$BMI = WEIGHT_{(pounds)} / [HEIGHT_{(inches)}]^2 \times 703$$

For example, if your weight is 200 lbs. and your height is 72 inches (6 feet), then your BMI should be $200/(72)^2 \times 703$ that is 27. Now, is that good or bad?
We can find that out in the following chart:

| BMI | Designation by WHO |
|---|---|
| Less than 18.5 | Underweight |
| 18.5- 25 | Normal |
| 25-30 | Overweight |
| 30 or more | Obese |

So, according to this chart, provided by World Health Organization (WHO), you will be considered as overweight.

- BMI does not take your muscle mass and body fat into account, so if you are a 90 kg athlete with low body fat then you will fall into the "overweight" category. So BMI is effective for an average person with an average muscle mass but once your muscle mass increases, the BMI is worthless. You can have a very good muscle mass and a fat percentage of 10 percent and still fall in the obese category.

- BMI is a good parameter for endomorphs trying to lose weight and track their progress. It is also good for ectomorphs as they are at times too skinny and help them analyze their weight   gain.

## Muscle Mass

Muscle mass varies from person to person. There are no ideal values for muscle mass in reference to height. It largely depends on a person's physical activity and his body type. For example a mesomorph person usually has a higher muscle mass than an ectomorph person. And a person, who exercises regularly, has a greater muscle mass than a person with a sedentary lifestyle.

## Weight for height

It is also an easy parameter for assessing a person's status of health. This is also most widely used parameter because everyone can interpret that from a simple chart.

| | Female Height to Weight Ratio | | | | Male Height to Weight Ratio | | |
|---|---|---|---|---|---|---|---|

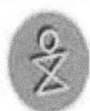

| Height | Low | Target | High | Height | Low | Target | High |
|---|---|---|---|---|---|---|---|
| 4' 10" | 100 | 115 | 131 | 5' 1" | 123 | 134 | 145 |
| 4' 11" | 101 | 117 | 134 | 5' 2" | 125 | 137 | 148 |
| 5' 0" | 103 | 120 | 137 | 5' 3" | 127 | 139 | 151 |
| 5' 1" | 105 | 122 | 140 | 5' 4" | 129 | 142 | 155 |
| 5' 2" | 108 | 125 | 144 | 5' 5" | 131 | 145 | 159 |
| 5' 3" | 111 | 128 | 148 | 5' 6" | 133 | 148 | 163 |
| 5' 4" | 114 | 133 | 152 | 5" 7" | 135 | 151 | 167 |
| 5' 5" | 117 | 136 | 156 | 5' 8" | 137 | 154 | 171 |
| 5' 6" | 120 | 140 | 160 | 5' 9" | 139 | 157 | 175 |
| 5' 7" | 123 | 143 | 164 | 5' 10" | 141 | 160 | 179 |
| 5' 8" | 126 | 146 | 167 | 5' 11" | 144 | 164 | 183 |
| 5' 9" | 129 | 150 | 170 | 6' 0" | 147 | 167 | 187 |
| 5' 10" | 132 | 153 | 173 | 6' 1" | 150 | 171 | 192 |
| 5' 11" | 135 | 156 | 176 | 6' 2" | 153 | 175 | 197 |
| 6' 0" | 138 | 159 | 179 | 6' 3" | 157 | 179 | 202 |

# Chapter 3

## What's Your Goal?

You should know your goals and what you have to do to achieve this goal and what's your gameplan.

➤ If you are an ectomorph with a BMI less that 20 then you should make a plan to gain muscle mass. To achieve this goal you should increase your intake of calories in the form of carbs and proteins (calorie surplus). Alongside that, you should do a moderate amount of cardio (not too much though). In this way, these carbs and proteins will be directed to muscle building in the body while maintaining a low fat percentage. You should do hypertrophy training and increase your muscle mass without accumulating fat.

➤ If you are an overweight endomorph with a high body fat percentage, you should plan to achieve two targets to reach your goals. 'Decrease your fat and increase your muscle'. You should target a calorie deficit and do a higher amount of cardio. This will help you lose body fat. Strength training is also advisable.

➤ If you are a mesomorph with a normal BMI, it is easier for you to achieve a lean aesthetic body. You have to lose the body fat by eating a moderate calorie diet and cardio and then monitoring your body fat percentages. You should increase your muscle mass by doing strength training.

Monitor your progress at regular intervals and make plan for your next step.

# Always Document, Control and Adapt

Let me give you some tips related to strength training. These small things will always help you in your goals.

- Always make a plan before doing anything. Do not start anything without a plan or you'll end up in a confused state. Plan every step of your training.

- Always document parameters related to your training, for example, calculate your BMI and measure your weight after regular intervals and note them regularly. In this way, you will have an idea in what direction you are going and if there is an improvement or not.

- If at some point, results are not coming then change the plan sensibly. Adapt to the new plan, document everything and track your progress.

- Do not lose hope at any time. Once you make a plan, you have got to follow it. I am telling you, 'it takes time'. You will need a higher level of strength and determination to do this. As the time passes, results will definitely start to come and your confidence will be increased.

## So, let's start

There are two domains of strength training. One is the 'Nutrition' part and the other is the 'Training' part. One cannot go without the other. Nutrition provides strength and energy to the body and Training directs this energy towards gaining muscle mass.

# SECTION - I
## <u>NUTRITION</u>

Nutrition is the source of energy for everything we do in our daily life. Seriously, everything, even reading and thinking requires energy. Most of our energy is consumed by the muscles during activity. When we use a muscle excessively and set the right kind of stimuli, it requires more energy from food and then this muscle starts to increase in size after getting that energy. So, a high quality and balanced food intake is crucial for building muscle mass.

I recommend a natural plant-based diet plan for athletes. The reason for this is it has a number of health benefits.

# Chapter 4

## <u>Benefits of Plant-based diet for Athletes</u>

Plant-based diets have hundreds of health benefits, proved by a large number of researches worldwide. One of the obvious reasons to adapt vegan diet is that it is more natural for our body's anatomy and it does not contain the health hazards associated with animal diet. A few reasons for athletes to plant based vegan diet are as follows:

- Athletes having a total plant based diet have **increased endurance** which in turn leads to a better performance.

- It is easier for vegan athletes to **have an ideal weight** because they avoid calorie dense foods, such as animal fats and dairy products. They consume high fiber and low calorie plant based diet which helps them in maintaining the ideal weight.

- Meat consumption increases the acidic levels inside the body, which favors inflammation and delay healing process. On the other hand, a plant based diet is usually alkaline in nature and **improves the recovery**.

- Plant based diets contain high amounts of anti-oxidants which decrease the lipid oxidation and prevent the cholesterol from clogging the blood vessels. Hence a vegan diet keeps you clean from the inside by **preventing cholesterol buildup.**

- Plant based diets provide an **easy physique maintenance** because unlike meat, it contains lesser fats. This makes it easy to maintain an aesthetic physique.

- People who consume a plant based diet have **reduced risk of diseases** including diabetes, hypertension, heart attack, obesity and some type of cancers. So, apart from providing improved athletic endurance, plant based diet also improves generalized health.

# Chapter 5

## <u>What are Calories and BMR?</u>
## <u>Why are they Important?</u>

**Calorie** (Kcal) is a unit of energy. It is widely used for calculating energy provided by certain foods.

After digestion, the food particles get mixed in blood and are distributed to almost every part of the body. At cell level, they get metabolized and then converted into energy. This energy is required to perform all the functions of the body. Interestingly, most of this energy is used to run the body's metabolism, which keeps the body warm all the time. Then comes the muscular activity and then all the other functions.

Extra energy is stored in the form of fat cells. This is why, when a person eats a lot, fat starts to accumulate in his body as storage. This storage gets used when a person starts calorie deficit.

## BMR

Basal metabolic rate (BMR) is the rate of energy spent per unit time at rest. For example, if you are just sitting down doing nothing, the energy expenditure rate during that time depicts your BMR. For some people BMR is high and for some people, it is lower.

People with high BMR tend to be ectomorphs because they have a high metabolic rate and a lot of their energy is spent in the process of metabolism. Reverse is true for endomorphs i-e low BMR

### Normal Daily Caloric Requirement

It is the precise number of calories required to perform daily normal function. It depends on a number of factors including your BMR, age, gender, height, weight and more importantly, your lifestyle. It gives an estimate of daily caloric energy, your body needs. It can be roughly determined from this table

Daily calorie needs based on age, gender, and activity level

| Age (Years) | Gender | Sedentary (Not Active) | Moderately Active | Active |
|---|---|---|---|---|
| 2-3 | Male or female | 1,000 | 1,000 | 1,000 |
| 4-8 | Male | 1,200 – 1,400 | 1,400 – 1,600 | 1,600 – 2,000 |
|  | Female | 1,200 – 1,400 | 1,400 – 1,600 | 1,400 – 1,800 |
| 9-13 | Male | 1,600 – 2,000 | 1,800 – 2,200 | 2,000 – 2,600 |
|  | Female | 1,400 – 1,600 | 1,600 – 2,000 | 1,800 – 2,200 |
| 14-18 | Male | 2,000 – 2,400 | 2,400 – 2,800 | 2,800 – 3,200 |
|  | Female | 1,800 | 2,000 | 2,400 |
| 19-30 | Male | 2,400 – 2,600 | 2,600 – 2,800 | 3,000 |
|  | Female | 1,800 – 2,000 | 2,000 – 2,200 | 2,400 |
| 31-50 | Male | 2,200 – 2,400 | 2,400 – 2,600 | 2,800 – 3,000 |
|  | Female | 1,800 | 2,000 | 2,200 |
| 51 and older | Male | 2,000 – 2,200 | 2,200 – 2,400 | 2,400 – 2,800 |
|  | Female | 1,600 | 1,800 | 2,000 – 2,200 |

Adapted from US Department of Agriculture and US Department of Health and Human Services. *Dietary Guidelines for Americans, 2010.* 7th ed. Washington, DC US Government Printing Office 2010.

# Track your Progress

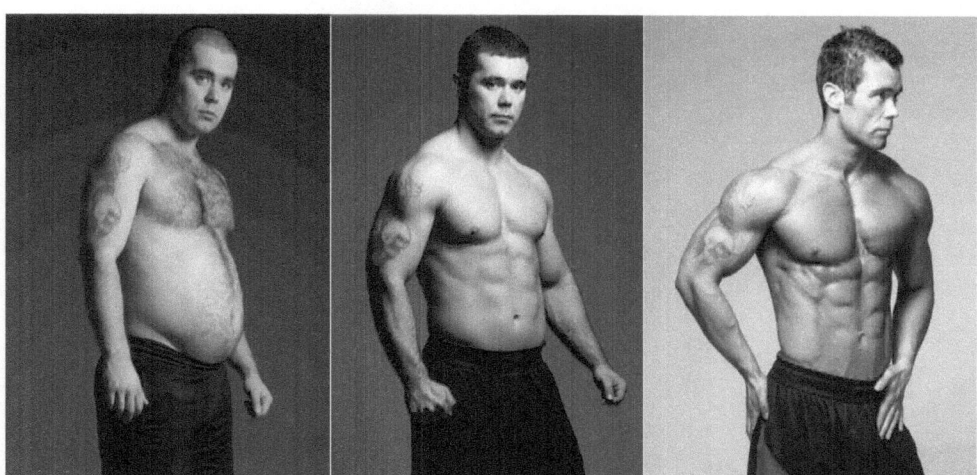

The most important thing in any type of training is to track your progress. Which way you are directed and whether you are improving or moving backwards or standing stationary. There are many ways to track your progress in strength training.

➢ The easiest method to track yourself is to look in the mirror every now and then and honestly assess your body. You can also assess your body by the way your clothes fit and what people say and comment about your body. Most people take pictures of themselves in the mirror at regular intervals.

➢ An accurate and simple way to measure your body composition especially fat composition is to do Anthropometric measurements of the body by a measuring tape. Document every time you measure your body composition. You can also make a chart to thoroughly track your progress.

➢ Regular measurement of body fat percentage gives you a good idea about your progress. This is most effective for endomorphs trying to lose weight.

➢ Calculating BMI is also a good and commonly used method, but it can be confusing because it does not take the muscle mass and body fat into account. It just compares your weight according to your height. It is a good method for endomorphs and obese trying to lose weight.

➢ Track your workouts and keep a record of every exercise you are doing. Write every exercise down including reps and sets. For example if you did 3 sets of 10 pushups last week for a total of 30 pushups, you need to be able to do 31 total pushups this week to be stronger.

# Chapter 6

## How to Get the Good Macros in

Macronutrients are the type of nutrients, which are required by the body in large amounts. ('macro' means large). These provide energy to the body for growth and daily activities.

There are three macronutrients,

Carbohydrates

Proteins

Fats

Now, I will explain, each one of them in detail and then mention the foods in which they are abundantly found.

- ## What are some Good Carbohydrate Sources

  Carbohydrates, also called carbs are one of the major sources of energy for human body. They are usually present in most of the things we eat. One gram of carbohydrate yields almost 4 calories of energy.

  ### Foods

  *Grain and rice are the most common forms of carbohydrates consumed. Carbs are also present in All the Green and Leafy **Fresh Vegetables**, Salads, Tomato, cucumber, Onions, Carrots, Beet, lettuce. **Fresh Raw Fruits** especially Apples, Oranges, Strawberries, Watermelon and Cantaloupe, Bread, Brown rice, Whole Wheat Bread, Oatmeal, Squash.*

- ## Foods that Contain Good Fats

  Fats are the most notorious of the macronutrients. One gram of fat yields about **9** Kcals of energy, more than double of what carbs provide.

  Fats have a lot of important jobs to do in your body. It helps in the absorption of certain vitamins into the blood strteam from your digestive tract, i-e vitamins A, E, K, D (fat soluble vitamins).Therefore, total fat restriction is not advised, as it can cause vitamin deficiency.

Fats found in vegetable and seed oils like **Omega 3 fats** increase the HDL in comparison to LDL. It means that they are good for the body because they increase the good lipoproteins and decrease bad lipoproteins. Research also proves that omega 3 fats are helpful in preventing cancer.

Fat is also responsible for hormone production and storage. For example testosterone is produced by estradiol inside fat cells. Many other hormones are also stored in fats.

So a normal and healthy intake of good fats is highly advised.

## Foods Sources

*Fat is found in vegetable oils, coconut oil, canola oil, seed oils, olives and olive oil etc.*

*Nuts, Flax seeds, walnuts and chia seeds are rich in omega 3 fats.*

## Indications for body types

Ectomorphs can take a good quantity of fat, but they should mainly refer to carbs for energy resources. They should take high amounts of good fats (high HDL). Mesomorphs should limit their fat intake to a minimum level, just to avoid the deficiency of fat soluble vitamins. They should rely more on good fats and avoid cholesterol containing fats.

Endomorphs should minimize their fat intake to only good fats (omega 3) and completely avoid the bad fats.

# • Proteins

Proteins perform a number of functions in the human body, including maintaining structure, growth and cellular signaling. Enzymes and hormones are also proteins. Proteins play an important role in building and maintaining the parts of the body, rather than providing as an energy reserve.

One gram of protein yields **4 calories** of energy, but this energy is mainly used for structural and functional role, rather than energy production.

Therefore, protein food is very important in the field of strength training, because the same proteins molecules we consume go and make up the muscles of the body and provide strength and endurance.

➤ **Average daily requirement** or recommended dietary allowance of proteins is 0.8g per kg of body weight or 50-60 grams for an average man. But if a person is an athlete or doing strength training then, his daily protein requirements is much higher than this level. Studies show that it raises up to 1.2 to 1.8g per kg of body weight or more than 80 grams per day.

➤ There are a lot of myths and misconceptions about vegetarian diets. Some people think that a plant based diet cannot fulfill the daily requirements of proteins. But the truth is, vegans can obtain sufficient amounts of amino acids from the vegetables and vegetable products.
    Let me prove that:

➤ As described earlier, an average person needs 0.8 grams per kg proteins per day and an athlete or bodybuilder needs approx. 1.2 grams per kg. Let say that a bodybuilder weighs 165 pound or 75 kg then, he will need only (75×1.2) **90** grams of proteins in a day. Yeah! You heard that right, 90 grams only. It's not that much if you consider that only 100 gramms of lentils provide you with up to 26 gramms of protein.

## Protein sources

The protein containing foods ranging from Non calorie dense to calorie dense are as follows:

*Low calorie protein foods include tofu, tempeh, soy beans, chickpeas, spinach, lentil, hummus, pita etc..*

*Calorie-Dense protein foods have both high calories and protein content. Examples are Quinoa, Amaranth, nuts like Hazelnuts, Chestnuts, Walnuts, Pine nuts, Peanuts, Pecans, Almonds, Black Walnuts. Seeds including Sesame, Hempseeds, Squash, Safflower, Pumpkin, Sunflower and Watermelon seeds. Nut butters specially Peanuts and Almonds, Beans, Soy Products, Soy cheese, Pea protein*

You can also make smoothies and protein shakes using pumpkin seeds, rice, hemp and peas, flaxseed, almond butter and chia seeds. I usually make a blend of any three or four of them in the morning, which gives me over 20 grams of protein in the start of the day.

Other great ideas for a good high-protein breakfast include **ALMOND BANANA CREAM SHAKE,** which provides a delicious and protein rich food in the very start of the day.

# Chapter 7

## Micronutrients are Important too!

Micronutrients are the type of nutrients, required by the human body in smaller amounts, throughout their life, to perform specific physiological functions. (micro means small).

Micronutrients are just as important as macronutrients. There are two main types of micronutrients: vitamins and minerals.

### Food Sources

Micronutrients are the organic compounds which are essential for the body and must be a part of our daily food intake. Common food sources for each vitamin include

- Green leafy vegetables, legumes, beans, pulses, potatoes, grains

- Superfoods

- Fruits especially citrus fruit like oranges, guava

- Seed oil, nut oil or simply nuts are also a very good food source of vitamins.

- Fortified granola cereals, beans and

# Chapter 8

## <u>Eat What Your Body Needs</u>

### (Food Sources According to Calorie Density)

I have listed a number of food sources classified according to the calorie density, from calorie dense foods to low calorie foods. Don't worry about making complex diet charts and following them. Just figure out a plan according to your body type and consume the foods that are best for your body. Keep the overall caloric intake in mind.

- **Calorie-Dense foods** are the best way to achieve calorie surplus for skinny people who are trying to bulk up.

  *Examples are nuts like hazelnuts, chestnuts, walnuts, pine nuts, peanuts, pecans, almonds, black walnuts. Seeds including sesame, Hemp seeds, squash, safflower, pumpkin, sunflower and watermelon seeds. Nut butters specially Peanuts and Almonds, Beans, Soy Products, Soy cheese, Pea protein, bulgar, quinoa, hummus Grains, Whole Wheat Bread, Pasta, Quinoa, Amaranth, Maize, Sweet Potato, Yams, Rice, Oats, Dried Apricots, Sesame Butter, Raisins, Dates, Honey, Dried Fruits and Dextrose, Fruit juices including Grapes, Pineapple, Apple and Orange juice*

- **Non Calorie- dense foods** are for those people who want to lose weight. Consuming non calorie dense foods is the best way to achieve calorie deficit.

  The examples are *tofu, tempeh, soy beans, chickpeas, spinach, lentil, , pita, kale, seitan, sunflower seeds*

  *Fresh Vegetables, Salads, Tomato, cucumber, Onions, Carrots, Beet, lettuce, Fresh Raw Fruits especially Apples, Oranges, Strawberries, Watermelon melon and cantaloupe contain more carbs and less caloric, Low Calorie White Bread, Brown rice, Whole wheat bread, Oatmeal, Squash*

You can choose from these foods, depending upon your body type and body needs.

Make sure to keep a track of your overall calorie intake.

Detailed food sources recommended for each body type are given in the following table;

| | Calorie-Dense Foods | Non Calorie-Dense Foods |
|---|---|---|
| **Carbohydrates** | **Calorie-Dense Carbs**<br><br>**Grains**, Whole Wheat Bread, Pasta, Quinoa, Amaranth, Brown rice, Whole wheat bread, Oatmeal, Squash<br><br>Sweet Potato, Yams, Rice, Oats, Dried Apricots, Sesame Butter, Raisins, Dates Honey, Dried Fruits and Dextrose<br><br>**Fruit juices** including Grapes, Pineapple, Apple and Orange juice | **Non Calorie-dense Carbs**<br><br>All the Green and Leafy **Fresh Vegetables**, Salads, Tomato, cucumber, Onions Carrots, Beet, Maize<br><br>**Fresh Raw Fruits** especially Apples Oranges, Strawberries, Watermelon, Melon and Cantaloupe contain more carbs and less calories |
| | **Calorie-Dense Proteins**<br><br>**Nuts** including Hazelnuts, Chestnuts, Hickory Nuts, Walnuts, Pine Nuts, Peanuts, Pecans,<br>Almonds, Butternuts, Beechnuts, Black | **Non Calorie-Dense Proteins**<br><br>Legumes: Lentils, Beans, Pita, Kale, Spinach, Peas, Broccoli, Seitan, Sunflower Seeds Corn And Popcorns |

| Proteins | Walnuts And Ginkgo Nuts, Dried Apricots, Dried, Oats, Bulgar, Quinoa, Hummus, Pea Protein **Seeds** like Sesame, Hemp seeds, Safflower, Squash, , Pumpkin, Sunflower And Watermelon Seeds **Nut Butters** Specially Peanuts And Almonds, **Beans,** Soy Products | Unsweetened Soy Milk, Tofu, Tempeh, Chickpeas, Kidney Beans, Pulses, Spinach |
| --- | --- | --- |

# Chapter 9

## The Effective Guide to Lose Weight

## (Say Goodbye to Extra Fat!)

Now, I will give a short and simple guide for weight loss. This is mainly directed towards endomorphs, overweight and obese people.

So, let's cut to the chase. There are two basic components of weight loss: Consuming lesser calories that is dieting and burning more calories that is exercise. These are really the only two ways to lose weight! Don´t believe in any fancy fat burning products, they are simple a scam.

### *Knowing your Calorie maintenance level*

Every person needs a certain amount of calories to perform his/her daily bodily tasks; it is called calorie maintenance level. It depends on your age, weight, height, BMR and most importantly your lifestyle. It is lower for a person with a sedentary lifestyle and much higher for an active person like an athlete.

On average, a person's calorie maintenance level is around **2500** calories per day. But, why am I telling you this?

**"The key to weight loss is that always keep your actual calorie intake below your calorie maintenance level"** This is called **Calorie Deficit.**

For example, if a person's daily calorie maintenance level is 2500 then, he should try to eat consume 2100 calories per day. This 400 calorie difference will be filled by the stored fats in your body.

## Calorie Deficit

For effective weight loss you should cut **300-500 calories** below your maintenance level. The best way to maintain this calorie deficit is eating non calorie dense food. Consuming Non calorie dense foods reduces your calorie intake below the maintenance level. This calorie deficit will make you lose weight. But, the question is, where should all your calories be coming from? What to eat and what not to eat?

## What to eat?

In general, you should focus on **Non Calorie dense foods** like fresh vegetables, fruits, soy products, pulses, tofu, tempeh, soy beans, chickpeas, spinach, legumes, beans and omega 3 containing fats.
Some people give strict charts to follow but my opinion is to eat smart. Here are some handy tips:

Eat fresh vegetables to help you feel full.

Drink a lot of water.

Get tempting foods out of your home.

Keep yourself busy -- you don't want to eat just because you're bored.

Don't eat while standing in front of fridge.

Don't skip meals.

Drink lots of green tea

## What not to eat?

This is more important than the previous section because these are the things that made you fat the first time. Basically, most of the processed food have a lot of low quality calories and many micronutrients removed and it is nearly impossible to achieve a calorie deficit while consuming them.

In addition, there are general types of foods you should also avoid to the specific items listed above, there are also certain types of foods that should also be avoided or at least limited. They are:

Foods containing high amounts of sugar

Foods high in saturated fat.

Foods containing any trans-fats

Foods high in sodium

# Burn more calories (Exercises):

No one needs to tell you that you should exercise regularly. Want to know why? Here are some benefits of regular exercise.

- It burns your calories. As I already described, it is helpful for weight loss. It's also helpful for avoiding weight gain. (7000calories deficit equals nearly 1kg body fat burned)
- It improves your physical abilities including strength,, flexibility and endurance. It makes you active and lively. It also makes you feel fresh
- It increases your muscle mass
- It improves your general health. It prevents a number of diseases including heart attack, diabetes, hypertension and high cholesterol etc. It is proved by a number of researches.

  In general, there are two types of exercises: aerobic exercise and anaerobic exercises.

## Do a lot of Cardio!

Cardio, which is short for cardiovascular, is also referred to as Aerobic exercise. This is called cardio because it increases the heart rate and improves blood flow through the body. These exercises are performed for longer periods of time and they provide cardiovascular endurance. This provides a number of health benefits. Some common examples of this type of exercise include

- Walking (At least for one hour daily)

- Jogging (Start slowly)
- Treadmill/ Elliptical trainer
- Swimming (Best for every muscle)
- Skating
- Biking (My favorite)

## Anaerobic Exercises

Anaerobic exercises are those activities that focus on increasing muscle strength. Anaerobic activities are performed for shorter periods and at high intensity, unlike aerobic exercises. Some examples include:

Resistance Machines

Weight Training

Calisthenics (pull ups, pushups etc.)

Since you are aiming to lose weight, you may be wondering why I would even bother doing an anaerobic exercise. Well, the answer is, it improves muscle strength, flexibility, bone density and the overall look of your body. The other main benefits are that the activity itself burns a lot of calories and it gives your body a very good shape.Having more muscle mass means a higher basal metabolic rate overall. So you burn more energy all the time so its harder to gain weight!

But if you are an obese person, you should first focus on losing the body fat through cardio and after you´ve lost a certain amount of fat, you should grow muscle mass by anaerobic exercises.

# Chapter 10

## How to Bulk Up Fast?

### (*A Fitness Trainer's Guide for Increasing Muscle Mass*)

Men find it very difficult to bulk up and gain muscle mass. The main reason for this is they are following the wrong advice. An advice that is not appropriate for their body. Most of the people end up following a program that is not even crafted for their own body type. Therefore, you need to follow a custom crafted program, specific for your body type.

## Bulking up requires a "Calorie Surplus"

To actively gain muscle mass, you need to create a net surplus of calories over time. Most people make a mistake at this point, that they do not eat enough, in accordance with their body type. If you want to gain and maintain a quality muscle mass, you should maintain a daily surplus of **250-500 calories** over a period of time.

### Calculate your calories

There are a number of formulas that you can use to calculate your calories precisely, for example the Harris-Benedict Equation, but to keep things simple try using the equation below:

Calorie intake = Body weight (in pounds) x 15 + 500 (surplus)

So, for an average 150lb man: 150 x 15 = 2,250 +500 = **2,750** calories

### Macros

Now, to achieve these calories, I recommend spliting your macros in the following way

Carbohydrate (70%) = 1925 calories/ 4 = 481g

Protein (20%) = 550 calories/ 4 = 137g

Fat (10%) = 275 calories/ 9 = 30.5g

# Recommended Foods

Now that we know the numbers, the next challenge is to decide about consumption. Generally I recommend mesomorphs to eat 2-3 meals per day, but ectomorphs are looking for extra muscle mass and size, so, it may be beneficial to spread the meals to about **5-7 meals** throughout the day. It will help ectomorphs combat their higher metabolic rates.

Let's move on to the choices of food. I recommend eating a wide variety of wholesome foods to counteract your high metabolic rates.

- **Protein sources** for ectomorphs include **calorie-dense** proteins like quinoa, lentils, pea protein, rice, hemp seeds, nuts and nut butter specially peanuts and almonds. I recommend a complete vegan diet, because it is completely natural and has higher health benefits.

- **Carbohydrates** should be consumed in the form of slow digesting food that will make you feel full. The examples include sweet potato, yams, quinoa brown rice and oats. But if you want to eat around workout time, it should be fast digesting foods because they can yield a higher amount of energy in a shorter time. Examples of fast digesting carbs include dates, honey, maize, fruit juices and dextrose.
- Good healthy **fats** are present in avocados, nuts, vegetable and seed oils, nut butters and coconut oil.
- Ectomorphs usually face trouble in eating high caloric meals throughout the day, so the solution to this problem is to take **liquid meals.** For example, I like to make healthy smoothies from simple ingredients like honey, oats, fruits and peanut butter. This is a blend of all the healthy ingredients and it should be taken before the start of training.

# Improve with Every Workout

Another rule of bulking is lifting heavier weights, because you are consuming a large number of calories and you have to channel that energy towards your muscles. It ultimately causes hypertrophy of the muscles.

- **Organize your training** into three phases, each phase lasting for four to six weeks. First, try to achieve a moderate muscle growth, and then progressively move towards higher intensity, such that your muscles are fatigued at the end of last repetition.
- **Improve your form** as you move forward. Perform each exercise to attain the maximum benefit out it and avoid injury.
- **Increase your Rep Range:** Increase the number of sets and reps to increase overload on your muscles which will lead to adaptation and hypertrophy.
- As you move forward, **lift heavier weights**. Always work with a spotter when you are lifting maximal free weights. You need to warm up thoroughly for 15 minutes by doing light exercises.

# SECTION - II
## Training

*The purpose of this section is to give you an overview and understanding of the common methods and terminologies used in strength training. So, let's start with the warm up exercises.*

# Chapter 11

## How to Warm-up Effectively?
## Why is this Important?

Every round of strength training starts with a good warm up. Warm up exercises have numerous benefits. I personally recommend a warm up exercise for every part of the body. Some people may undermine the importance of warm up exercise but they are very important because:

➤ Warm up exercises increase the temperature of the body and prepare it for maximum performance.
➤ When the muscles are stretched and twisted during warm up, their elasticity is increased.
➤ Warm up exercises increase the heart rate and heart pumps more blood and nutrients throughout the body.
➤ Warm up exercises also improve the body's range of motion.
➤ Warm up exercise generates a higher energy level, which stimulates the release of hormones.
➤ Warm up exercises prepare athletes mentally for their raining.

### *Some examples of warm up exercises*

Some people think that walking and running is the only warm up exercise necessary, but I recommend that you should choose warm ups that can cover almost every part of your body and prepare most of your muscles for the high intensity training.

➤ **Workout with lighter weights**

In my opinion, the best way to warm up is doing the same workouts with lighter weights. The reason is that the muscles are prepared for the high intensity training individually.

➤ **Pushups**

Pushups are an important warm up exercise before any type of workout. You should do five to ten pushups before starting your workout. It makes your heart pump more blood towards your upper body. Therefore, it prepares your body for the heavy weightlifting.

> **Cardio**

Running or jogging is the basic warm up exercise. It makes your body warm in general and increases the pumping activity of the heart that increases the blood flow to every part of the body. So, always take two or three rounds of a nearby park, or run on a treadmill for five to ten minutes.

> **Warm up your rotator cuff**

The rotator cuff is the socket of your shoulder girdle. In order to warm up your rotator cuffs you have to warm up the muscles around your shoulder girdle. Prepare your shoulder with 4-5 light exercises which may include front and lateral raises, shrugs, bicep curls and lateral rotations. The details are mentioned in the exercise catalog. These exercises warm up your shoulder girdle and get it ready for the heavy lifting because most of the weight is transferred through this region.

> **Twist your upper body**

When you twist your upper body, your abdominal muscles undergo a certain amount of stretching. Make sure to twist your upper body in every direction. For example, put both your arms on your hips and then twist the upper part of your body, first to the right and then to the left.

> **Move your limbs**

Limbs are the main parts of the body to do most of the heavy lifting, all four limbs should be moved in every possible direction. Make sure to move your arms in both clockwise and anti-clockwise direction. This will also prepare you mentally for the training.

> **Make your own warm up**

Basically, warm up is any exercise that increases your body temperature by generating heat from the muscles. Every muscle should be warmed up individually. You can also try the following exercises

Skipping, Knee lifts (30 times in 30 seconds), Knee bends (ten times), Shoulder rolls

(2 sets with 10 repetitions)

You can also make your own type of warm up exercises, the point is, you just have to make your muscles undergo a quick and light phase of activity, that will prepare your body for high intensity exercise.

# Chapter 12

## The Basic Techniques of Strength Training

Strength Training is a type of physical exercise in which a person contracts his muscles against an increasing resistance, which progressively increases the size, strength and anaerobic endurance of the muscles.

Strength training has a number of significant health benefits which include giving strength to the ligaments and muscle tendons and improved joint motility and function, increased metabolic rate, increased bone density, improved heart function, lower LDL (Bad cholesterol) and increased HDL (Good cholesterol) and increased general body fitness.

## General Technique of Strength Training

Strength training involves the manipulation of an increasing number of exercises, repetitions, sets, resistance, force and tempo to bring about the desired muscular hypertrophy.

The specific combination of reps, sets, exercises and resistance should be different for every person.

- The science behind the technique of strength training is that it increases the force output of muscle, progressively by increasing the weights. It also uses certain equipment and exercises to target specific muscle groups. Basically, it is a rule of nature that, when you increase the activity of a muscle, it starts to increase its size and strength in response. This increase in size and strength of muscles is called **"Hypertrophy"** So, in short, the purpose of the training is to simply overburden the muscles with extra load and in response to that it increases in size.

- It necessitates that training of each muscle group should be synchronized with other muscle groups, like chest/biceps/shoulders. To achieve a maximum training effect, the lifts should be done with heavy weights (70 to 80% of 1RM i-e HIT) and multiple sets and there should not be la too long resting period in between the sets (2 to 5 minutes on average) depending upon the intensity of the training.

- The effectiveness of this training lies in the fact that each muscle group should be challenged sufficiently and the threshold of the overload should be reached. The overload should be increased gradually sothat the muscles will ultimately grow.

# Some terminologies you need to know

There are several specialized terminologies that are used to describe the parameters of strength training.

### Form

It is a specific way to perform the movements of a training exercise to maximize the benefit of the exercise and avoid an injury and prevent cheating.

### Rep

It is the shorter form of repetition. One rep represents a single cycle of lifting up the weight and then lowering it down, moving through the form of an exercise in controlled manner.

### Tempo

It is defined as the speed with which a training exercise is done. The tempo of an exercise can affect the strength of a muscle and it differs with the weight a person is handling.

### Set

Set means, several repetitions performed in a continuous sequence with no break between the repetitions. The number of sets per exercise and the number of repetitions performed in a set totally depend on a person's goal, as to what extent he wants to gain muscle mass.

### RM

Rep maximum or RM is defined as the maximum number of repetitions, a person can perform for a given weight. For example, if a weight is so heavy that you can only perform one rep with it then the RM for that weight would be 1RM.

If you can perform 8 reps with a weight of 80 pounds, then your RM for that weight would be 8 RM.

# Chapter 13:

## <u>What is Split Training?</u>

Split training targets certain muscle groups at a time. And then focuses on another muscle group at a different day.

Split training can be divided into different types of routines - one of them is push/pull/legs split and the other one we are going to mention is a upper body/lower body spit.

- In **Push/Pull/Legs Split** the body is divided into three groups of muscles, push muscles, pull muscles and legs. A push workout is the one that requires you to push weight for example seated presses and barbell bench presses and triceps push down. Whereas pull exercise require you to pull the weight against the resistance, for example seated cables rows, sit up, standing calf raise and barbell curl are pull exercises. Legs workout will train the entire lower body.

  Push muscles of the upper body include Chest, Triceps and Shoulder. Pull muscles include Biceps, back muscles and Abdominals. Legs workout will include Quads, hams and calves.

  In this routine, you divide your week days for push and pull exercises alternatively and ultimately covering your whole body.

  A classic sample for 7 days cycle of **push/pull/legs routine** is as follows:

  ➢ Day 1: Push Workout (Chest, Triceps, Shoulders)
  ➢ Day 2: Rest
  ➢ Day 3: Pull Workout (Back, Biceps, Abs)
  ➢ Day 4: Rest
  ➢ Day 5: Legs Workout (Hams, Calves, Quadriceps)
  ➢ Day 6: Rest
  ➢ Day 7: Rest

Note that the rest days are as important as the workout days because the muscles do not grow during exercise periods, they grow during the rest or recovery period. So, you need to give them proper time for rest so that hypertrophy can occur.

- Talking about **Upper/Lower Split,** as the name depicts, you divide the body in upper and lower parts. Upper body muscle groups include Chest, Triceps, Shoulders, Back and Biceps and lower body muscle groups include Calves, Quadriceps, Hamstrings and Abs. You train your upper body on one day and your lower body on the alternate day. A sample of upper/ lower split routine is as follows

  - Day 1 : Calves, Quadriceps, Hamstrings, Abs
  - Day 2 : Chest, Triceps, Shoulders, Back, Biceps
  - Day 3 : Rest
  - Day 4 : Calves, Quadriceps, Hamstrings, Abs
  - Day 5 : Chest, Triceps, Shoulders, Back, Biceps
  - Day 6 : Rest
  - Day 7: Rest

# Chapter 14

## <u>What is The Best Workout Routine?</u>
## <u>How to decide?</u>

There are hundreds of workout routines out there, but what will be best for you... This can be a very frustrating question. It starts with whether to choose a full body training program or a split training program?

- As we have already discussed, a split training routine means that you have divided your muscle groups in Upper/lower or Push/pull/legs and you alternate them throughout the week with rest days in between.
- In contrast to that, full body routine is the type of workout in which you train your entire body and all the muscle groups on the same day with alternating rest days.

### Factors That Decide Your Best Routine

Most people choose a training routine by idealizing a successful and advanced athlete and blindly following his routine but it most often is the wrong approach.

The question here is that "What is the most optimal and best workout routine?" The honest answer to that question is that there is no "best" workout routine out there. You cannot generalize one training routine to everyone. It all comes down to your personal preferences.

*Your best workout routine depends on your goals, experience, progression and your schedule.* You have to consider all these factors before choosing a workout routine. So, we will discuss every one of these and how they affect your workout routine.

> ### ➤ Your Goal decides your routine

Your workout routine mainly depends on your goals and what you want to achieve with your body. Do you want to build muscle or lose fat? You want to become stronger or do you need more endurance? All these things determine your best workout routine. If you want to build more muscle mass, choose a routine that gives maximum hypertrophy. Do a sports specific training if you want a sprinter's body. Your goals should be in line with your training.

## ➢ What's Your Experience Level?

How long have you been working for? Are you a beginner or an intermediate or an advanced builder? What is your experience level? A lot people tend to set their experience level much higher than they actually are and this is not a good approach. If an intermediate level athlete starts working on an advanced level routine, he will not get the optimal benefits from that. Just because anything sounds more complex does not mean it will be beneficial for you. Similarly, if you are a beginner, do not run towards the intermediate programs. They are not designed for your level. Follow a program that is created for the beginners. Develop your form, learn how to do a specific movement, find out your biomechanics and leverages. Develop a strength base and a foundation for yourself and then gradually move to another level of experience.

## ➢ Keep Your Schedule In Mind:

Don't make a routine that conflicts with your schedule like work, school or social life. Choose a routine that is the best fit for your schedule. Most of the people can only go to the gym three days a week realistically but they go ahead and choose a program that requires them to attend six days a week. This is a mistake and would cause trouble in both training and social life.

## ➢ Progression

Progression is the key to any successful program. You have to make sure that you are progressing otherwise there is no point in training. A lot people go to the gym daily and they try all the routines and work very hard but they don't make any progress because they don't choose a progresive routine.

So, pick a routine that promises some built-in progression and some improvement over time.

# Chapter 15

## A Comprehensive Guide to High Intensity Interval Training (HIIT)

### What is HIIT?

High intensity interval training (HIIT) is also called Sprint interval training (SIT) or High Intensity Intermittent Exercise (HIIE). It is a modern form of interval training in which short and intense periods of anaerobic exercise are altered with lesser intense periods of recovery. It is a type of cardiovascular exercise. A session of HIIT may vary from five to thirty minutes. These short and intense periods of anaerobic exercise provide improved calorie expenditure and fat loss, improved glucose metabolism and a good athletic condition and capacity to the body.

- A single session of HIIT starts with a warm up exercise, which is followed by 3-10 repetitions of high intensity exercise. These repetitions are separated by recovery periods of medium intensity exercise. Then, it is ended with a cool down exercise. Almost maximum intensity is used in high intensity exercise and almost 50% intensity is used in medium intensity interval.

- The length and number of repetitions varies with each exercise, therefore there is no specific regimen for HIIT. It totally depends on a person's capability and stamina and cardiovascular development. Usually a 2:1 formula is used. For example 50 seconds of high intensity workout (sprinting) is followed by 25 seconds of slow walking.

- It is good to keep a timer or watch with you and constantly note the time intervals of every phase of training. A typical session of HIIT can vary between five to thirty minutes.

## Why should you do HIIT?

High intensity interval training has a number of benefits for the body.

- HIIT is one of the most efficient forms of cardio and it doesn't require equipment and a lot of time in the gym.

- It burns huge amounts of fat. Some experts say that HIIT burns six times more fat than general cardio. So this is excellent for weight loss

- It increases your metabolic rate and doesn't let your metabolism slow down, which in turn increases the expenditure of calories

- It increases muscle size and strength tremendously. The muscles grow in a shorter period of time.

## When Should You Do HIIT?

- HIIT Training is a great alternative to regular cardio training. If you want to get ripped or simply want to loose weight, HIIT is a great solution.

- People usually tend to do HIIT on the rest days but my recommendation is to do it right after their weight lifting session. I do not recommend people to do it on non-weight lifting days because I like to keep them 100 percent rest days.

- In the beginning, do HIIT just two times per week on non-consecutive days. Give your muscles rest for at least 48 hours between sessions so they can repair and grow stronger. As you become stronger, add in a third session per week if you desire.

- Limit your HIIT workouts to no more than 3 times per week. Do not try to do more, especially if you're doing heavy lifting since this will most likely lead to overtraining.

# A Basic program for HIIT

If you are a beginner, then the following program can make you an advanced athlete in an about eight to ten week time.

**Phase 1 (Week1-2)**

The work to rest ratio in this phase is 1:4 and the total training time is about 15 minutes. Its duration is from week 1 to week 2.

➢ High intensity exercise for 15 seconds

➢ Rest or low intensity exercise for 60 seconds

Repeat this process another 10 times, and then end the session by doing a final high intensity blast for 15 seconds.

**Phase 2 (Week 3-4)**

In this phase, time of high intensity exercise is increased and the work to rest ratio climbs to 1:2. As a result, the total time of workout climbs up to 17 minutes. Its time frame is from week 3 to week 4.

➢ High-intensity exercise for 30 seconds

➢ Rest or low-intensity exercise for 60 seconds

Repeat this process another 10 times, and then end the session by doing a final high intensity blast for 30 seconds.

**Phase 3 (Week 4-5)**

In this phase, the rest interval is reduced to half and now the work to rest ratio is 1:1. And the total duration of workout is 18.5 minutes. The time frame of this phase is from 5-6 weeks.

➢ Rest or low-intensity exercise for30 seconds

➢ High-intensity exercise for 30 seconds

Repeat this process another 11 times and end the session by doing a final high intensity blast for 30 seconds.

**Phase 4 (Week7-8)**

In this phase, the rest time is finally reduced to half and the rest ratio becomes 2:1. The time duration in this phase is 20 minutes. By the time you reach this phase, you will become an advanced level athlete.

➢ High-intensity exercise for 30 seconds

➢ Rest or low-intensity exercise for 15 seconds

Repeat this process another 25 times and end the session by doing a final high intensity blast for about 30 seconds.

You can improvise and change the time according to your will. For example if you think that a particular phase is getting too easy for you then you can move up to the next phase. Similarly, if you think that you should spend some more time in a particular phase then you can spend more than two weeks. So, improvise sensibly.

## Exercises

You can do following **exercises** in High intensity interval training after a general warm up and stretching.

Pushups for 3 minutes (45 second: work and 15 second rest), Pull ups (3 rounds: 45 seconds work and 15 seconds rest). Same thing can be done with Squats and Triceps dips. There is a one minute recovery period after every round. Others exercises include: High Knees - 25 yards, Touch Toes - 15 reps (Touch toes quickly, come right back up and repeat), Arm Circles - 20 reps, Lunges - 10 reps/leg, Side Lunges - 10 reps each direction

| Did you Know? |
|---|
| A muscle does not actually grow during the exercising period. It increases its size during the resting/recovery period. Therefore resting intervals are as important as high intensity periods. |

# Chapter 16

# The Basics and Benefits of Circuit Training

Circuit training is a form of workout in which resistance training and body conditioning are done using high intensity aerobics. An exercise "circuit" refers to completion of all the given exercises in a workout program. When one circuit of exercises is complete, the next one begins from the first exercise of the circuit. Typically, the time interval between the exercises of a circuit is short and the person moves rapidly towards the next exercise in the circuit. It promotes muscular endurance and strength building.

## Typical exercises in a circuit

The following exercises can be used in a circuit training session

Upper body: Bench dips, Press ups Pull ups, Bench lift, Medicine ball chest pass, Inclined press up

Core and trunk: Back extension chest raise, Stomach crunch (upper abs), Sit ups (lower abs)

Lower-body: Bench squat, Hopping shuttles, Shuttle runs, Step ups

Total body: Skipping, Squat thrusts, Treadmills, Burpees

## Examples of circuit training session

In order to give you the concept of circuit training, here are some examples of circuit training sessions.

### With 6 Exercises

You should do all of the following exercises in a circuit with minimum rest periods between any of the two exercises.

- Suspended Row
- Romanian Deadlift

- Loaded Pushups
- Trap Bar Deadlift
- Chin up
- Goblet Squat

For all these exercise, do 1 set with 5 reps. Repeat the circuit for five times.

## With 8 exercises

- Back extension,
- Shuttle Runs,
- Bench Dips,
- Squat Thrusts,
- Sit ups,
- Squat jumps,
- Press ups,
- Treadmill

## Duration

Work on each exercise for 20-30 seconds and take resting time of maximum 30 seconds between two exercises. Do 5 sets of each exercise and maximum resting time should be 3 minutes.

The whole training should consist of a four week cycle. This four week cycle should comprise an easy week, a medium week, a hard week and a test/recovery week. You can improvise the workload by changing the number of sets, reps, duration, resting time and even exercises. You should choose the circuit that best fits your body.

## Pros

Circuit training has the following advantages

- You have plenty of exercises to choose from
- All the exercises are easy and simple
- Flexible routine and scheduled and the exercises can be changed according to fitness and age of athlete
- It develops an athlete's endurance and strength

## Cons

The circuit training has following disadvantages:

- Many exercises require special gym equipment.
- It can be expensive and a lot of space is also required to set up the equipment.
- The equipment may need a level of expertise, training and safety monitoring.

# Chapter 17

## Six Effective Compound Exercises for MASS BUILDING

How to build some serious muscle mass? How to make your body "big" in the gym? The best way to achieve these goals are compound exercises. Compound exercises are the ones that involve more than one muscle group and more than one joint.

***Compound exercises are one of the best ways to gain and built muscle mass. (Check out:*** *THE SUPER SIX WORKOUT: DISCOVER THE PROVEN MOST EFFECTIVE EXERCISES TO PACK ON SERIOUS MUSCLE MASS QUICKLY by Scott Oteri on Amazon for more Information on these specific exercises and an advanced training program.)*

According to my recommendation, the following six exercises are the best compound exercises out there. These exercises give great results in building muscles, and they normally cover all of your body. A brief overview of each of them is given here. Refer to "The Exercise Catalog" for more details.

# 1. Squats

Squats are the best exercise if you want big legs and a strong back. For this exercise, imagine yourself as if you are sitting in an invisible chair. Doing this exercise with the right technique is very important.

This is one of the best compound exercises that uses just about every muscle in your lower body as well as many on your upper body. Primarily it works your Quads and secondarily it targets Hamstrings, Back, Calves, Gluts, Abductors and Adductors.

## 2. Deadlifts

This exercise focuses on building the thickness of mid to lower back. It also develops overall strength in the body as it is very much a whole body exercise involving legs, back, shoulders, arms and Calves. The main muscles involved in deadlifts are Lower Back muscles. Others include Calves, Quadriceps Hams, Gluts, Latissimus dorsi, middle back, Traps and forearms

In terms of workout economy, deadlifts get a lot of work done in a very short space of time because to some extent, almost every muscle of the body gets used.

## 3. Bench press

Bench presses are one of the most commonly performed exercises in the gym today. Beginners love to perform this exercise and it is usually an important part of routine for almost every exercising athlete. It is a horizontal pushing exercise and targets most of your upper body pushing muscles. Bench press involves the Pectoralis Major primarily. It also works your anterior Deltoids and Triceps Brachii muscles secondarily. Bench presses are the best exercise to make gains in the chest and shoulder area in a short time.

## 4. Military Press

If you want to get thick and wide shoulders then this is the best exercise for you. It is best done with a barbell. It is also called overhead press or shoulder press.

Primary target muscle of military press are the Deltoids. It also works your Triceps, Pectoralis Major and Latissimus Dorsi muscles indirectly.

## 5. Pull Ups

This is one of the most popular upper body exercises and rightly so. It is the best compound exercise for shoulders and back. Target muscles are Latissimus Dorsi (Lats), Deltoids, Biceps and middle back. Wide, medium and narrow grips can be used but wide grip is mostly recommended because it emphasizes more on the lats muscle and helps you get a V shape to your back.

## 6. Bent Over Rows

Bent over row gives you a very strong back. This compound exercise can be performed with either a narrow grip or a wide grip. Each variation works your muscles in a different way therefore the grip decides the target muscles. Wide grip targets the muscles across the back of your shoulders specifically your posterior Deltoids, Trapezius and Erector Spinae. Narrow grip mainly targets Latissimus Dorsi (lats). Both these grips involve Biceps, lower back and legs to more or less the same degree.

*So, if you have to choose, these 6 exercises are the best compound exercises. These simple exercises are easy to incorporate into your schedule and they are very effective in building muscle mass.*

# Chapter 18

## What are Isolation Exercises?

## How to decide your Isolation Exercise ?

Isolation exercises are those exercises, which target one muscle group and one joint instead of multiple joints and muscles as compared to compound exercises. Isolation exercises let you take care of each individual muscle group. These exercises are the best way for training in detail.

- In my opinion, the best approach is doing both the isolation and compound exercises in a combination, according to the preferences of your body. This will give you more control over each part of your body and you can pay attention to any particular muscle group of the body. For example, if you think a muscle is lagging behind in your compound exercise routine then you can start isolation exercise for that particular muscle.

- Some isolation exercises according to muscle groups are the following:

  - Abdominals:   Decline crunch, Cable crunch, Oblique crunch
  - Back:   Straight Arm pull down, Incline Bench Pull
  - Biceps:   Barbell Curls, Dumbbell Curl, Hammer Curl
  - Chest:   Cable Crossovers, Butterfly
  - Triceps:   Extension, Pushdowns
  - Shoulder:   Lateral Raise, Front Dumbbell raise (Deltoids)
  - Calves:   Raise, One legged Cable
  - Hamstrings:   Lying Leg Curl, Standing Leg Curls
  - Quadriceps:   Leg Extensions

### How to Decide Your Isolation Exercises?

In my opinion, add some isolation exercises to your compound exercise workout routine. You should be fine with 1-3 isolation exercises per workout. Keep in mind, that you should focus on getting stronger at the compound exercises, as they are the ones mainly responsible for muscle growth. Improvise, according to your body and decide your own isolation exercises. For example, if you think that your Deltoids are weaker and are lagging behind in your compound workout routine, then you should add Lateral Raises to your routine.

The details of these exercises are mentioned in the exercise catalog.

# Chapter 19

## **Principles of Weight Training:**

If you hit the gym daily but just lift every other weight blindly then you will end up nowhere. There is a certain set of rules that must be followed to gain the maximum results out of strength training. After reading these rules, you will be able to figure out you own program and you will have a good plan of action.

- **Selection of Exercise:** Choose your exercise wisely. Select those exercises which are optimal for your body. My suggestion is choose certain compound exercises (that involve more than one joint and muscle group) and add just one or two isolation exercises (that involve one joint and muscle group) according to your body requirement. For example if you can´t keep a good form performing your squats because your knees move inward, add abductor exercises to your routine. This can vary from person to person, so look at your form and choose your isolation exercises smartly.

- **Number of Sets:** Choosing the number of sets is quite crucial and will ultimately depend on the intensity level you are working with. You will learn more about the number of sets in the training programs later on.

- **Number of Reps:** Be careful while deciding number of reps per set. It depends on your basic fitness level, your goal, age, body type and your experience level. Keep all these factors in mind while deciding. Low number of reps (2-5) per set develops strength and has no impact on endurance. 8-12 reps per set will increase the muscle size (hypertrophy). More than 13 reps per set increase anaerobic endurance.

- **Frequency of Sessions:** The effectiveness of a training workout program depends on two things; the intensity of the exercises and the time management of the exercises. The time management includes the rest periods too. Resting periods are as important as the higher intensity period because the resting periods allows the muscles to recover and give them time for adaptation and hypertrophy. It is important to plan each day of your routine and frequency of your workout sessions. If your goal is endurance, you have to increase the training sessions per week to about 8-12. If you want strength, training session frequency should be 3-6 per week and if you want hypertrophy it should be 5-7 sessions per week, with appropriate rest periods in between.

- **How much Load**: Selection of a proper weight for an exercise depends on the total number of reps, sets, form and intensity of that particular exercise. Take the moderate approach for hypertrophy. Increase the load to 80-90 percent, if you want to increase strength and take it to 40-60 percent if your goal is endurance.

- **Rest between Set**: Rest for 2-4 minutes between the sets if you want hypertrophy and strength. Take it to 1-2 minutes if you want endurance. If you decrease the resting period between the sets, your body will pull energy from the anaerobic system which in turn will eventually result in increased anaerobic endurance.

| Variable | Training goal | | | |
|---|---|---|---|---|
| | Strength | Power | Hypertrophy | Endurance |
| Load (% of 1RM) | 80-90 | 45-60 | 60-80 | 40-60 |
| Reps per set | 1–5 | 1–5 | 8–12 | 13–60 |
| Sets per exercise | 4–7 | 3–5 | 4–8 | 2–4 |
| Rest between sets (mins) | 2–5 | 2–5 | 2–4 | 1–2 |
| Duration (seconds per set) | 5–10 | 4–8 | 20–60 | 80–150 |
| Training sessions per week | 3–6 | 3–6 | 5–7 | 3–10 |

# Chapter 20

# <u>How to Break Plateaus;</u>
# <u>Training Periodization</u>

Training Periodization means to plan your training routine systematically in order to avoid overtraining and get the required results. It includes the cycling of various aspects of your training progressively throughout the year. Here we will divide the whole year into smaller periods/phases and set aims for each of these phases. Each phase ends with a specified goal/target.

If you don't use periodization, what usually happens is that your body copes with your style and intensity of training and adapts to it, achieving a plateau. After that, it stops showing progress regardless of your regular training. ***Periodization never lets your body achieve a plateau*** and ensures a continuous growth of your body.

There are some specific terminologies which are used to describe the training periodization. These are the phases of periodization which have a single goal by the end of that training period.

## <u>Macrocycle</u>

Macrocycle is a 52 week *annual plan* that is directed towards a goal towards the end of the year. It guides an athlete's training throughout the year and is designed to achieve the peak performance. It includes all four stages of a training program (**intensity**, **endurance competition** and **recovery**). It can be further divided into different phases including preparatory phase, competitive phase and transition phase.

## Mesocycle

Mesocycle is a shorter part of the macrocycle, which consists of two to six weeks. During a mesocycle, one aspect of training is prioritized and when that aspect is achieved, the next mesocycle begins. It may vary, depending on the type of training. A bigger plan is divided into smaller plans which are achieved in smaller time periods (mesocycles).

For example if you want to achieve hypertrophy of a muscle group at the end of a mesocycle, you should do 4-8 sets with 8-12 reps for 4-8 weeks. During a mesocycle, a single aspect of training is emphasized.

## Microcycle

Usually, a microcycle spans about a week. Microcycle is a part of mesocycle, which in turn is a part of macrocycle. A microcycle is planned in such way that it gives an athlete a way to adapt to his training sessions. This planning is usually done at the weekly level. For example if you are training three days a week, you could use the first two days to build up to a third 'heavy day' when you will train at a high intensity. When an athlete stops making progress or successfully adapts to the training program then some changes to the training variables are made and the next microcycle begins.

## An example of Training Periodization:

If you are a beginner, this is how you can apply the training periodization in your routine. During the first phase of 2-3 months, lift heavy, do a lot of compound exercises like squats, bench press, military press. This is the *hypertrophy phase*. Your muscles will suddenly feel stress and will respond by hypertrophy.

The next phase is *transition phase*. Once you have bulked up a bit, you can go easy on the compound exercises in this phase. Add some isolation exercises in your routine accordingly. You can also do "weak point training" during this phase in which you give special attention to the weak part which was not hit by the compound exercises. For example if you have a strong chest and weak legs. Go easy on the chest exercises a bit and add leg curls and squats to your routine.

The last phase is *light period* of 4 weeks in which you go even lighter on isolation exercises and do more cardio to burn some extra fat. You will have a "ripped look" at the end of this phase.

# Chapter 21

## <u>How to have a Stronger Mind with a Strong Body: The Mental Game</u>

If you want to change your body and lifestyle at a bigger level, you must change your mental attitude. If your mind isn't ready to change then it's very difficult to complete the job because your body will never be up to the task in that case.

The mental game has a pivotal role in achieving your goal, whether it is losing weight, gaining muscle mass or getting lean or all of them! All these physical things are controlled by your mind. If you read the biographies of the great achievers in every sport, there will be one thing they will have in common, and that is *a strong mental game*. They achieved everything by being on top of their mental game. Therefore a strong mental game can be the difference between success and failure.

The work, you have to do in strength training can be tough and hectic sometimes, so you will really need a very strong attitude for that. *You can't get away with a weak mental attitude in strength training even if you are an advanced athlete.*

You can make anything happen by improving your mental strength. Here are a few changes that you should bring to your mindset in order to have a stronger mental game.

- ### *<u>Know your goals</u>*

  You have to know your goals before starting any program. It is your body and you should know what you want to do with it. Whether you want to bulk up or you want to get lean. Whether you want a lot of muscle mass or you want the body of a sprint athlete.

  Whether you want to become a professional fitness model or you just want to remain fit. *Always keep your target in mind*. You should also know that in which direction you should move. Otherwise you will only wander off in different directions and end up nowhere.

Use your mind before determining your goal; otherwise it may cause havoc. For example, if a person, who is already overweight, decides to gain a lot of muscle mass, it's not a good idea for him. His first goal should be to lose fat first and then gain muscle mass.

Once you have determined your goal sensibly, stick to it and don't let it go, results will come, *I assure you they will*. There will be a lot of obstacles in your way trying to derange you from your path. **Even your family and friends might not support you** and they might criticize you on spending too much money and time on your goal. You should not let them move you from your path; instead you should take them into confidence and try to gain their support.

- ### *Do whatever it takes*

You have to do whatever it takes to achieve your goal. You have to do what you hate, even more than usual. For example, if you don't like doing lunges, do even more. If you don't like your diet, eat more foods without spices. It you hate doing cardio; increase the speed and time of treadmill. **Fight your weaknesses and fight them in such a way that they should not remain your weaknesses anymore**.

Do all the hard stuff with joy and interest. It will ease your daily routines and it will make other tasks of your life look easy. If you are doing the hard stuff easily then all the other stuff won't be a problem for you anymore.

So, always remember this principle: **If you feel that something is too hard for you; do it even more!** Even when you are outside the gym, it is a good thing if you follow these rules there too. You have to incorporate this principle to every aspect of your daily life.

- ### *Create positive energy around you*

When you start a program to change your body shape, you may find a lot of people around you that may discourage and criticize you. **They may call you obsessive or even mad**. This may distract you from your goal and hinder your progress. Believe me, this is a lot more common than you think. At first, you may not be affected but as the time passes, this constant negativity will bring you down and will affect everything you are doing.

The key to a successful workout program is creating a constant positive atmosphere around you. This is encouraging and supportive for you and you will move towards your goal easily.

If there are a lot of negative people around you, don't let them influence you in any way. So, **the key is to simply avoid negative people**, who discourage you, even if they are your friends.

Similarly, it is also important to surround yourself with positive people, the people, who always encourage you. If you are mostly alone, then spend more time with other athletes and lifters who are just as dedicated as you. This way, you will get a constant encouragement from a constant example around you.

- ## *Don't Lose Momentum*

Strength training, like any other habit, is very tough to start. But once it starts, it is much difficult to break. On the other hand, *if you break the streak, it is very difficult to restart.* So once you start, keep it up. Don't let your routine break and don't let your inner laziness overcome your spirit.

You should try to make your routine tight at present so that you could feel relaxed with it tomorrow. Once you make a routine regarding diet, sleep or work, your mind and body will become familiar with it in a short span of time. If you break the routine, all that familiarity will be lost. So you should try to make a balanced routine which is based on your determination. At beginning it will make you feel uncomfortable and can also affect your temper but you should fight it. Soon your body and mood will become familiar with it.

Next time, you are thinking of skipping a workout, ask yourself; is it worth it? Should you break your momentum for such a trivial thing? So, don't make a bad decision at that time or you'll suffer in the future.

The moral of the story is that, stick to your healthy diet and complete your workout regularly. It will benefit you in the long run. **Make this apparently "tough" routine your natural routine**. Once the improvement begins, you will love the direction you are going and you will hate going back to the unhealthy, weaker and smaller version of yourself.

- ### *Accept the failures*

  *No matter how much you try to make it right, you will certainly have setbacks in your training*, and they can come from anywhere. For example external stress, injuries, low energy periods and missed workouts. You may lose your heart during the training period, especially when the results are not coming. You just have to keep looking for the best direction and if you are in the right direction already, then keep going. Believe me you will get the desired results someday. Just don't lose your focus.

  *You have to fight every setback that comes in your way*. Make time for the gym; don't let yourself eat a lot, try positive reinforcement. You can't deny occasional setbacks, there has to be a setback after some days. You just have to make it right by *optimizing everything in your control*. Just have the right mind set and you will bounce back on the right track.

- ### *Set smaller goals*

You should have two types of goals in your mind; short term and long term goals. Most of the people have long term goals in their mind but the question is how to achieve it? My bet is by setting smaller goals that lead to it.

For example, if a person is overweight and he wants to become a fitness model, he has to *split it up into smaller goals*. He should first lose body fat and then try to gain muscle mass by full body or split training and side by side he has to modify his diet too. All these are smaller goals. By achieving these smaller goals step by step, he will achieve his big goal.

Let's take another simple example. Let's say you are doing 100 lunges in five reps and you want to take this number to 200. You have to split it up into smaller goals. First, get to 120 then 150, then 170 and then 200. It will make your bigger goal a lot easier.

# Chapter 22

## How To Get A Six Pack

### *(Myths And Mistakes)*

Six pack a fantasy or a reality? For some of the people, this is really a fantasy but since I tend to live in a real world and see people having ravishing six packs I am inclined to say that it is a very attractive reality.

It is a reality that people want to look attractive and want to attract others with their figure and physique but many things come in their way. There are many factors, rather facts which come in their way.

### What Is A Six Pack?

Six pack is a sheet of muscle called "rectus abdominis" which extends from ribcage to the pubic bone. It is supported by internal obliques, internal obliques and erector spinae with which it provides support to our spine and our vital for sports activities. Abs specific exercises to develop six pack should cover this whole area. These exercises do not only make our bodies attractive but also help us stand tall and perform better in everyday activities.

### Everyone Has Six Packs

After reading this line, you must have looked at your abdomen and wondered if I am kidding but actually this is true. Everyone has six packs. It is basically a sheet of muscle called rectus abdominis, as mentioned earlier, present in the abdominal wall. The problem is that in majority of the cases, it is covered by large deposition of fats between six packs and skin that's what hides it. The way to have six packs visible is through well planned workout and proper diet. Most of the times, you don't even have to train your abs isolated or with specialized exercises. The main focus should lie on proper diet changes to lose that fat layer.

## Laziness Is The Key To Uneven Body

One of the factors which hamper appearance of six packs is laziness. It is well documented that a very small percentage of people have the tendency to attend the gym in order to achieve bodily fitness, for the lazy ones it is like a dream they can never achieve and they are quite content with their lives on sofa accompanying chips and dip in front of a television.

## No Plan, No Gain

One of the greatest problems I see among the people who fail to make six packs visible is the lack of a proper plan and guidance. It is often seen in gyms that many people who are inspired by some good looking actor or a well-shaped wrestling superstar are in hurry to acquire ideal shape. In this hurry, and without proper guidance, they start doing some very strong exercises as if they want to have abs by the time they leave the gym that day. What happens next? The enthusiastic exerciser gets severely cramped up and is not able to even leave his bed. This puts a very bad impact on the aim of a good shaped body and it gradually fades away.

## What To Do To Have A Six Pack?

In order to be able to six pack appear, a well guided plan is necessary which should comprise of following steps.

**Set an achievable goal:** The goal should be moderate and not to be intense as it will decrease compliance to the plan. Remember, the key to good shaped abs is consistency.  Don't be over ambitious

1. **Diet:**

   Diet should be modified and this modification should be done while keeping in mind that we need to burn the fat and need energy for building muscles. Carbohydrates are not bad so it is advisable to just let go the processed foods while enjoying the rest. Protein intake should be increased as more protein is required to build up muscles. Processed food and fast food meals should be avoided as they lead to fat accumulation which mainly starts in your belly. ***Calorie deficit and burning fat is more important for getting a six pack than exercises***. Keep good hydration and drink lots of water as it helps in body metabolism. Eat more non-calorie dense foods and never let stomach be empty so that stored energy does not get used.

2. **Exercise:**

The Workout should be started with an achievable plan starting with basic general workouts like the six compound exercises which work your abs enough. But if you want to move towards more specific isolated exercises targeting the core here are a few examples.

> **Specific exercises:** Some of the exercises which lead to good shaped abs with six pack include crunches, planks, bench leg raise, jackknife, barbell rollout, pike, pull up and increase in cardio.

> **Variations in exercises:** Exercises should be varied after sometime and if the body becomes too comfortable in an exercise, either change it or increase the force.

> **Priority of sequence:** If one thinks that his abs is the worst part of the body and needs more work out, then he should start his basic exercises focusing on the core since at that time the body is fresher and has more energy.

## A Moderate Plan For Six Pack

As discussed earlier, in order to get a proper six pack, a proper plan with guidance is necessary. This plan should begin with making some goals like how much weight you want to lose in one month and what you are going to do for it. This should be followed by diet modification focusing on losing fat and gaining muscle mass.

Perform minimum one set of each exercise three times a week as a beginner and aim for 8-12 reps in each set. Once these exercises become easy, add another set. These exercises include:

- **Cardio** to be done in intervals but should have high intensity. An interval can be as short as 30 seconds but the intensity should be high.
- **The bicycle** 2 sets of 12 reps are a good start.
- **Wood chop** 1 set of 12 reps is enough for beginners
- **The pike** one set of 8-12 reps as a start
- **Crunches** include many types like sided crunches, weight crunches etc. One set of any of these with 8-12 reps is sufficient for a beginner.
- **Pull ups** one set with 8-12 reps is enough for a start.
- **Ball slam** 3 sets of 10 reps each with 60 seconds brake in between.
- **Barbell rollout** 3 sets of 10 with 2 mins brake in between sets.

## How often should I be training?

The goal to achieve a perfect six-pack almost every time results in people trying to put extra effort on their core. These people think that extra effort may result in extra good but that is not the case as hitting their midsection hard after every workout may result in over training. The abdominals are just like any other muscle in the body. They also need some rest in between workouts. If rest is not given to the muscles, it will lead to constantly overworked state which would prevent better results. *The six compound exercises as mentioned earlier are best for strengthening abdominals.* These should be done with proper rest in between. Remaining exercises are designed for specific surrounding muscles and should be done to strengthen them respectively.

## What Not To Do? (Mistakes To Be Avoided)

- **Don't do too much** as it will lead to lots of fatigue and irritability and may lead to non- compliance.
- **Watch your diet** and avoid anything which increases fat.
- **Avoid infomercials** and their "quick result" equipment. Remember, key to six pack is consistency and there is no shortcut

- **Avoid starvation** as it may lead to usage of proteins from body and also decrease metabolism leading to lesser fat burning.
- **Avoid medication** like fat loss pills, steroids or muscle gaining medication as they may lead to more harm with their side effects than good results.

## Myths To Be Ignored

- You cannot have a six pack.
- Six pack appears overnight.
- Supplements will help a lot in getting a six pack.
- Only crunches result in six pack.
- You must leave carbohydrates alone.
- Once you get six pack, your work is done.
- I will get a perfect six pack like models.
- I do not need exercise if my diet is good.

# Chapter 23

## <u>Gain Strong Confidence With A Shredded Body</u>

Our appearances and bodily health affects our capability and confidence. A lean and healthy person most often has a higher level of confidence than an obese person.

### Problems with an obese person

It is justifiable to say that every person has a right to the way he wants to live. This world is equal for people of every kind belonging to any race, gender, ethnicity, religion or country. We, the social animals, are supposed to be social to others and follow this simple fact that every person has a right to live in his own way but we make a mistake and tend to forget it. We indulge ourselves in the matters of other people's lives and judge them according to their appearances and discriminate on its basis.

An obese person has to face criticism on almost everyday basis regarding his physique or how much unpleasant he is to others. People tend to limit their contact to people on the basis of pity reasons such as looks and appearances and tend to have more social contact with better shaped people. This not only leads to a limited social life of obese person but also has a very bad effect on his confidence.

### Confidence gains in person who starts working out

It is a known fact that greater one feels good about himself, greater he starts believing in himself. It can be visible from the people who have lost weight and have adapted to a much better looking shape with their utmost effort and consistency. Such people feel rewarded and feel that if they can change their appearance, they can change anything. Moreover, the fact that they are not being ridiculed in the society anymore due to their uneven appearance also leads to confidence building.

## A shredded person can shred anything

When a person knows he has power to do anything, has a perfect shape and a body to charm anyone, it automatically adds to the confidence of the person. He is seen as a role model by some members of the society like those who are trying to gain an ideal physique. Some people envy him and that adds up to the feeling that he is something. Girls are more attracted to such person and try to increase contact with him and this makes his confidence sky high because let's face it, body builders' dream always have the part where he is surrounded by beautiful girls who all just want to touch those tight abs (This might encourage the reader even more to start working for those abs much quicker and with more devotion). A person with such marvelous body has so much self confidence that he is not afraid to face any social situation. He is not afraid of any encounter because the feeling of having a good looking, rather ravishing personality brings something special out of him.

# Chapter 24

# <u>Training Programs to Achieve Strong Lean and Aesthetic Body</u>

If anyone decides to start bodybuilding, the biggest challenge is to find the best training program. It is crucial to find a good training program as it can effect one's progress. There are plenty of workout programs out there but it's hard to choose a single best plan.

I will first describe the program for beginners (program 1) and then for advanced beginners (program 2).

## <u>Program 1 (For the Beginners)</u>

This program is designed for the beginners. *This is a full body workout program* and it's best for those who just started doing workout. Full body workout starts up the whole body as it involves
training most of the muscle groups of the body on the same day.
Split body workout program is not appropriate for the beginners. It is recommended for advance beginners.

Just follow ***some basic rules*** before starting the program:

- Every major muscle group should get one exercise.
- The weights should be lighter during first two weeks because it is necessary to practice your form.
- Add another set in the weeks 3-4; also do a little warm up set before main exercise. The weights should be slightly heavier in this phase. Your muscles should be exhausted at last rep. Do not overdo anything or you will lose your form.

- During 5-8 weeks, do a good warm up set before starting and lift more challenging weights in this phase. It is better if you gradually increase the weights (lower the reps) towards the second and third set. Do not choose too heavy or too light weight. It should be optimum for you. Such that your muscles are completely exhausted after reaching the target rep.
- Now, I will describe an example of a *full body workout plan for beginners*. Note here that this program is just an example. Exercises, reps, sets, 1RM percentages are also mentioned.

  It should be followed *for six to eight weeks* and after that you can move to program 2, which is for the level of advanced beginners.

## Program 1 (Full Body Workout) For Beginners

|  | Week 1 | Week 2 | Week 3 | Week 4 | Week 6-8 |
|---|---|---|---|---|---|
| **Load (% 1RM)** | 65% | 65% | 70% | 70% | 70-80% |
| Squats | 2×15 | 2×15 | 3×10-12 | 3×10-12 | 3×8-12 |
| Leg Presses | 2×15 | 2×15 | 3×10-12 | 3×10-12 | 4×8-12 |
| Pull Ups | 2×15 | 2×15 | 3×10-12 | 3×10-12 | 3×8-12 |
| Bench Press | 2×15 | 2×15 | 3×10-12 | 3×10-12 | 3×8-12 |
| Seated Dumbbell Press | 2×15 | 2×15 | 3×10-12 | 3×10-12 | 3×8-12 |
| Triceps Dip Machine | 2×15 | 2×15 | 3×10-12 | 3×10-12 | 3×8-12 |
| Standing Barbell Curl | 2×15 | 2×15 | 3×10-12 | 3×10-12 | 3×8-12 |
| Machine Crunch | 2×15 | 2×15 | 3×10-12 | 3×10-12 | 4×8-12 |

- Some general principles for the beginner's program are as follows;

  **Training Frequency:** 3 days

  **Training Days:** Monday, Wednesday, Friday

  **Sets Per Exercise:** 2 to 3 sets

  **Reps per set:** 10-15

  **Rest Between Sets:** Up to 2 minutes

- When you finish a set, your muscles need some time to clear out the accumulated lactic acid. This can take from 60 to 120 seconds. So, you should *rest for up to 2 minutes* between the sets. The rest period depends on the intensity of exercise you are doing. The higher the rep range/lower the intensity, the less rest you need between sets of that exercise. The lower the rep range/higher the intensity, the more rest you need between sets of that exercise.

- These exercises should be performed 3 times a week on the non-consecutive days. This will allow your body to recover and let the adaptation process go on during the rest days.

Another good way to make your training program is to divide the exercises into A and B groups. Both have a different sets of exercises. Diversifying your workout will make it more fun and interesting.

> **Workout A:**

| | |
|---|---|
| Barbell Squats | 3 sets with 12-15 reps |
| Bench Press | 3 sets with 12-15 reps |
| Lateral Raises | 3 sets with 12-15 reps |
| Pull ups | 3 sets with 12-15 reps |
| Bent over Barbell Rows | 3 sets with 12-15 reps |
| Sit Ups | 3 sets with 12-15 reps |

## ➢ Workout B:

| | |
|---|---|
| Front Squats | 3 sets with 12-15 reps |
| Dead lifts | 3 sets with 12-15 reps |
| Push Ups | 3 sets with 12-15 reps |
| Military Press | 3 sets with 12-15 reps |
| Seated Triceps Press | 3 sets with 12-15 reps |
| Barbell Curls | 3 sets with 12-15 reps |

- Do these workouts on the three nonconsective days of the week, like ABA with rest days in between. This will cover all the regions of your body and you will achieve full body strength as the program moves forward.

# The Training Load Chart

| Max reps (RM) | 1 | 2 | 3 | 4 | 5 | 6 | 7 | 8 | 9 | 10 | 12 |
|---|---|---|---|---|---|---|---|---|---|---|---|
| % 1RM | 100% | 95% | 93% | 90% | 87% | 85% | 83% | 80% | 77% | 75% | 70% |
| Load | | | | | | | | | | | |
| 10 | 10 | 9.5 | 9.3 | 9 | 8.7 | 8.5 | 8.3 | 8 | 7.7 | 7.5 | 7 |
| 20 | 20 | 19 | 18.6 | 18 | 17.4 | 17 | 16.6 | 16 | 15.4 | 15 | 14 |
| 30 | 30 | 28.5 | 27.9 | 27 | 26.1 | 25.5 | 24.9 | 24 | 23.1 | 22.5 | 21 |
| 40 | 40 | 38 | 37.2 | 36 | 34.8 | 34 | 33.2 | 32 | 30.8 | 30 | 28 |
| 50 | 50 | 47.5 | 46.5 | 45 | 43.5 | 42.5 | 41.5 | 40 | 38.5 | 37.5 | 35 |
| 60 | 60 | 57 | 55.8 | 54 | 52.2 | 51 | 49.8 | 48 | 46.2 | 45 | 42 |
| 70 | 70 | 66.5 | 65.1 | 63 | 60.9 | 59.5 | 58.1 | 56 | 53.9 | 52.5 | 49 |
| 80 | 80 | 76 | 74.4 | 72 | 69.6 | 68 | 66.4 | 64 | 61.6 | 60 | 56 |
| 90 | 90 | 85.5 | 83.7 | 81 | 78.3 | 76.5 | 74.7 | 72 | 69.3 | 67.5 | 63 |
| 100 | 100 | 95 | 93 | 90 | 87 | 85 | 83 | 80 | 77 | 75 | 70 |
| 110 | 110 | 104.5 | 102.3 | 99 | 95.7 | 93.5 | 91.3 | 88 | 84.7 | 82.5 | 77 |
| 120 | 120 | 114 | 111.6 | 108 | 104.4 | 102 | 99.6 | 96 | 92.4 | 90 | 84 |
| 130 | 130 | 123.5 | 120.9 | 117 | 113.1 | 110.5 | 107.9 | 104 | 100.1 | 97.5 | 91 |
| 140 | 140 | 133 | 130.2 | 126 | 121.8 | 119 | 116.2 | 112 | 107.8 | 105 | 98 |
| 150 | 150 | 142.5 | 139.5 | 135 | 130.5 | 127.5 | 124.5 | 120 | 115.5 | 112.5 | 105 |
| 160 | 160 | 152 | 148.8 | 144 | 139.2 | 136 | 132.8 | 128 | 123.2 | 120 | 112 |
| 170 | 170 | 161.5 | 158.1 | 153 | 147.9 | 144.5 | 141.1 | 136 | 130.9 | 127.5 | 119 |
| 180 | 180 | 171 | 167.4 | 162 | 156.6 | 153 | 149.4 | 144 | 138.6 | 135 | 126 |
| 190 | 190 | 180.5 | 176.7 | 171 | 165.3 | 161.5 | 157.7 | 152 | 146.3 | 142.5 | 133 |
| 200 | 200 | 190 | 186 | 180 | 174 | 170 | 166 | 160 | 154 | 150 | 140 |
| 210 | 210 | 199.5 | 195.3 | 189 | 182.7 | 178.5 | 174.3 | 168 | 161.7 | 157.5 | 147 |
| 220 | 220 | 209 | 204.6 | 198 | 191.4 | 187 | 182.6 | 176 | 169.4 | 165 | 154 |
| 230 | 230 | 218.5 | 213.9 | 207 | 200.1 | 195.5 | 190.9 | 184 | 177.1 | 172.5 | 161 |
| 240 | 240 | 228 | 223.2 | 216 | 208.8 | 204 | 199.2 | 192 | 184.8 | 180 | 168 |
| 250 | 250 | 237.5 | 232.5 | 225 | 217.5 | 212.5 | 207.5 | 200 | 192.5 | 187.5 | 175 |
| 260 | 260 | 247 | 241.8 | 234 | 226.2 | 221 | 215.8 | 208 | 200.2 | 195 | 182 |
| 270 | 270 | 256.5 | 251.1 | 243 | 234.9 | 229.5 | 224.1 | 216 | 207.9 | 202.5 | 189 |
| 280 | 280 | 266 | 260.4 | 252 | 243.6 | 238 | 232.4 | 224 | 215.6 | 210 | 196 |
| 290 | 290 | 275.5 | 269.7 | 261 | 252.3 | 246.5 | 240.7 | 232 | 223.3 | 217.5 | 203 |
| 300 | 300 | 285 | 279 | 270 | 261 | 255 | 249 | 240 | 231 | 225 | 210 |
| 310 | 310 | 294.5 | 288.3 | 279 | 269.7 | 263.5 | 257.3 | 248 | 238.7 | 232.5 | 217 |
| 320 | 320 | 304 | 297.6 | 288 | 278.4 | 272 | 265.6 | 256 | 246.4 | 240 | 224 |
| 330 | 330 | 313.5 | 306.9 | 297 | 287.1 | 280.5 | 273.9 | 264 | 254.1 | 247.5 | 231 |
| 340 | 340 | 323 | 316.2 | 306 | 295.8 | 289 | 282.2 | 272 | 261.8 | 255 | 238 |
| 350 | 350 | 332.5 | 325.5 | 315 | 304.5 | 297.5 | 290.5 | 280 | 269.5 | 262.5 | 245 |
| 360 | 360 | 342 | 334.8 | 324 | 313.2 | 306 | 298.8 | 288 | 277.2 | 270 | 252 |
| 370 | 370 | 351.5 | 344.1 | 333 | 321.9 | 314.5 | 307.1 | 296 | 284.9 | 277.5 | 259 |
| 380 | 380 | 361 | 353.4 | 342 | 330.6 | 323 | 315.4 | 304 | 292.6 | 285 | 266 |
| 390 | 390 | 370.5 | 362.7 | 351 | 339.3 | 331.5 | 323.7 | 312 | 300.3 | 292.5 | 273 |
| 400 | 400 | 380 | 372 | 360 | 348 | 340 | 332 | 320 | 308 | 300 | 280 |
| 410 | 410 | 389.5 | 381.3 | 369 | 356.7 | 348.5 | 340.3 | 328 | 315.7 | 307.5 | 287 |
| 420 | 420 | 399 | 390.6 | 378 | 365.4 | 357 | 348.6 | 336 | 323.4 | 315 | 294 |
| 430 | 430 | 408.5 | 399.9 | 387 | 374.1 | 365.5 | 356.9 | 344 | 331.1 | 322.5 | 301 |
| 440 | 440 | 418 | 409.2 | 396 | 382.8 | 374 | 365.2 | 352 | 338.8 | 330 | 308 |
| 450 | 450 | 427.5 | 418.5 | 405 | 391.5 | 382.5 | 373.5 | 360 | 346.5 | 337.5 | 315 |
| 460 | 460 | 437 | 427.8 | 414 | 400.2 | 391 | 381.8 | 368 | 354.2 | 345 | 322 |
| 470 | 470 | 446.5 | 437.1 | 423 | 408.9 | 399.5 | 390.1 | 376 | 361.9 | 352.5 | 329 |
| 480 | 480 | 456 | 446.4 | 432 | 417.6 | 408 | 398.4 | 384 | 369.6 | 360 | 336 |
| 490 | 490 | 465.5 | 455.7 | 441 | 426.3 | 416.5 | 406.7 | 392 | 377.3 | 367.5 | 343 |
| 500 | 500 | 475 | 465 | 450 | 435 | 425 | 415 | 400 | 385 | 375 | 350 |

## How to Use Load Assignment Chart?

*You can estimate the amount of weight you can lift from this chart.* Say your 1RM for Squat is 270. You want to do a set of 10. You can consult the chart and know that 200 lbs. is the weight to use for 10 reps and this will 75 % of maximum intensity.

*The Load Assignment Chart is also useful for Estimating Your 1 Rep Max.* Say you squat 160 pounds and are just able to perform 8 reps before you cannot perform another rep. Find the 160 under 8 reps on the chart and follow the chart over to the left. Your 1RM would be around 200 pounds.

# Program 2 (For Advanced Beginners)

As you go through the program 1, your body will start to show improvement, your muscles will become stronger and bigger and you will gain weight. At this stage, when you have gained noticeable muscle mass and strenght, you can move from beginner to advanced beginner stage. (approximately after 10 weeks)

- The advanced beginner stage has a different set of exercises, with different intensity and routine. The full body workout program is changed to a **Split Training program**, in which each muscle group is trained on different days of a week. This is recommended for advanced beginners as they are ready to train their specific muscle groups after the full body workout in program 1.
- This is not recommended for beginners because their body needs full body workout to start up as a whole. After that, they can split up their body according to their own preferences.
- There are two ways to do split training. The body can be split up into upper and lower parts, or it can be divided according to push/pull/leg exercises.
- Keep in mind that these exercises are performed with a gap of at least one day. This day is the resting/ recovery period. Resting period is just as important as the workout period because *the muscles actually grow during the recovery period.*
- You can also add some isolation exercises accordingly. As you go through program 2, your body starts to reach the pro level gradually.
- **Training Frequency:** 3 days
  **Training Days:** Mondays (push), Wednesdays (pull), Fridays (legs)
  **Reps per set:** 5-10
  **Sets per exercise:** 3-4
  **Rest between Sets:** 2-3 minutes

The classic sample of program 2 is described below. Keep in mind that this just an example. You can improvise and add your own exercises according to your preferences and body requirements.

The routine for *Push/Pull/Leg split* is given below in the form of a chart.

# Table

| | Week 1 | Week 2 | Week 3 | Week 4 | Week 5 | Week 6 |
|---|---|---|---|---|---|---|
| **Program 2 (for Advanced Beginners)** **Push/Pull/Leg Split** | | | | | | |
| Load (% of 1 RM) | 80% | 80% | 83% | 85% | 85% | 90% |
| **Session 1- Push   (Mondays)** | | | | | | |
| Bench Presses | 3×6-8 | 3×6-8 | 3×6-8 | 3×4-6 | 3×4-6 | 3×4 |
| Barbell Shoulder Presses | 3×6-8 | 3×6-8 | 3×6-8 | 3×4-6 | 3×4-6 | 3×4 |
| Dumbbell Overhead Triceps Extension | 3×8 | 3×8 | 3×8 | 3×6 | 3×6 | 3×4 |
| Incline Dumbbell Flyes | 3×12-15 | 3×12-15 | 3×12-15 | 3×15 | 3×15 | 3×15 |
| Triceps Press Down | 3×12-15 | 3×12-15 | 3×12-15 | 3×15 | 3×15 | 3×15 |
| **Session 2- Pull   (Wednesdays)** | | | | | | |
| Lat Pull Down | 3×8-10 | 3×8-10 | 3×8-10 | 3×6 | 3×6 | 4×4 |
| Barbell Row | 3×6-8 | 3×6-8 | 3×6-8 | 3×6 | 3×6 | 4×4 |
| Seated Cable Rows | 3×12-15 | 3×12-15 | 3×12-15 | 3×15-20 | 3×15-20 | 3×15-20 |
| Barbell Curl | 3×6-8 | 3×6-8 | 3×6-8 | 3×4-6 | 3×4-6 | 4×4 |

| Barbell Shrugs | 3×6-8 | 3×6-8 | 3×6-8 | 3×4-6 | 3×4-6 | 3×4-6 |
|---|---|---|---|---|---|---|

## Session 3- Leg    (Fridays)

| | | | | | | |
|---|---|---|---|---|---|---|
| Squats | 3×6-8 | 3×8 | 3×8 | 3×4-6 | 3×4-6 | 3×4 |
| Leg Press | 3×6-8 | 3×6-8 | 3×6-8 | 3×4-6 | 3×4-6 | 3×4 |
| Lying Leg Curls | 3×12 | 3×12 | 3×12 | 3×15 | 3×15 | 4×15 |
| Standing Calf Raise | 3×20 | 3×20 | 3×20 | 3×25 | 3×25 | 3×25 |
| Leg Extensions | 3×12 | 3×12 | 3×12 | 3×15 | 3×15 | 3×15 |
| Crunches | 3 sets × max. rep | 3 sets × max. rep | 3 sets × max. rep | 3 sets × max. rep | 3 sets × max. rep | 3 sets × max. rep |

# Chapter 25

# <u>The Exercise Catalog</u>

Following the given guidelines and examples of workout programes, you should be ready to put together your own custom crafted program. Here are the most effective exercises to reach your goals!

## <u>Legs</u>

### 1. Squats

This is one of the basic exercises for your legs. This exercise should be performed carefully as there is a risk of injury. If you have some issues with your back then you should try some alternatives. If you have a healthy back then perform this exercise properly with extra care.

*Type: Compound Leg Exercise*
*Target Muscles: Quadriceps, Glutes, Adductors, Calves, Hamstrings, Hip Flexors, Abs*

- Get inside the squat rack and place the bar on the correct height around the level of your shoulder. Load the bar get under it, with your back of shoulder touching the bar.
- Hold the bar with your arms on each side and gently lift up the bar by pushing

your legs. Now, move a few steps away from the rack. Your legs should be positioned correctly with your toes slightly pointing outwards. Keep your back straight and your head should be upright.

- Start the exercise by gently lowering the bar by bending your hips and knees. Keep your head up, maintaining the straight posture. Keep going down until the angle between your thighs and legs is around 90 degrees. At this point, breathe in some air.
- Now, start going up gently as you exhale the air. Straighten your legs by pushing the floor.
- Repeat the process until the target number of repetitions is reached.

## 2. Front Squats

This is almost the same as the regular squats but the only difference is that the bar is held in front of your head instead of back of the shoulder. You will find it easier to have an upright upper body throughout this exercise than during the conventional Squats and Front Squats stress the Quads a little bit more!

*Type: Compound Leg Exercise*
*Target Muscles: Quadriceps, Glutes, Adductors, Calves, Hamstrings, Hip Flexors, Abs*

- Load the bar after choosing the correct height. Bring your arms towards the bar. Keep your elbows high. Put the bar on your deltoids while crossing your arms and grasp the bar with both hands.
- Rest of the steps is almost the same as regular squats. Step away, go down, inhale, move upward and exhale while maintaining the straight and head up posture.

- Repeat the process.

## 3. Leg Curls

*Target Muscle: Hamstrings*
*Type: Isolation Leg Exercise*

- This exercise can be done on a preacher bench or a lat pull down machine using their leg pads.
- Put your ankles under the padded lever. Put your knees on the seat and looking away from the machine. Maintain an upright posture.
- From this starting position, extend your knees slowly and under complete control, lower yourself to the ground and put your hands on the ground.
- Now, gently push the ground and lift yourself up, maintaining the control. Returning to the starting position.
- Repeat until you reach the target repetitions.

## 4. Leg Press

This exercise is done on a leg press machine. There are three foot stances, that can be used for this exercise but the most common stance is the medium stance or the shoulder width stance.

*Target Muscles: Quadriceps, Glutes, Adductors, Calves, Hamstrings, Hip Flexors*
*Type: Isolation Leg Exercise*

- Sit on the machine and put your legs on the platform of the machine. Remove the safety bars that hold the weight and then push the platform with your legs, all the way up, As far as your legs can go and fully extend. Do not lock your knee joint otherwise there will be no exertion.

- Your legs should make an angle of 90 degrees with your torso. Keep your legs fully extended. This is considered as your starting position.
- Take a deep breath and gently lower the platform until there is an angle of **90 degrees** between your thighs and lower legs.
- Now exhale and push the platform with your heels, going back towards the starting position. This movement will use your quadriceps.
- Repeat, until the desired number of repetitions is reached.
- Make sure to lock the safety bars before finishing the workout, otherwise, the loaded platform can fall on you.

## 5. Calf Raise

This is the best exercise for your calves. This is considered as an isolation exercise.

*Target Muscles; Gastrocnemius, Soleus (Calf Muscles)*
*Type: Isolation Leg Exercise*
This exercise can be done by two ways; seated and standing. Both of them are explained one by one.

**Seated Calf Raise**

This exercise works the Soleus muscle in your calf underneath gastrocnemius. When you are
seated, the Gastrocnemius is taken out of the movement due to the bent angle of the knee.

- Put your toes on the platform of the machine and extend your heels. You can use any toe position including forward, out an in.

- Adjust the lower pad according to the length of your thighs and put your lower thighs under it. Now put your hands on the lever pad. This will stop them from slipping.
- In order to get to your starting position, push your heels upwards, slightly lifting he lever and then remove the safety bar.
- By flexing your ankles, slowly lower your knees. This will stretch your calf muscles. Take a deep breath while doing this.
- Now, extend your ankles and raise the heels high in order to contract your calf muscles maximally. Exhale the air while doing this.
- Repeat until the desired number of repetition is reached.


**Standing Calf Raise:**
Calf raise can also be performed while standing. It can also be performed using barbell as well as dumbbell if the machines are not available. This exercise works your Gastrocnemius muscle
which is present on the back side of calf. So, apparently, both the calf raises may have the same
function, but you need both of them for full calf development.

- Adjust the lever of the machine according to your height.
- Facing your toes forward put your shoulders below the padded lever. By doing extension at knee and hip joint, push the lever upwards. Keep your torso straight. There should be a mild bend at your knees. Do not lock them. This is your starting position.
- Exhale and extend your ankles, raising your heels as high as they can go. Contract your calf muscles. Do not bend your knees and keep them steady. Stay in this position for at least a second.
- Now, lower the heels and start going back towards your starting position. Stretch your calf muscles and bend your ankles as you go back. Take a deep breath while doing this.

- Repeat this process until you reach the desired number of repetitions.

| DID YOU KNOW? |
| --- |
| The "**Soleus** Muscle" in your calves is also called Peripheral **HEART**, because it has venous spaces filled with blood. When this muscle contracts, it pumps the blood upwards. |

# Back

## 1. Pull Ups

There are certain types of grips for this exercise.

Wide Grip: is the one in which the distance between your hands is more than the width of your
shoulders. This grip emphasizes more on the latissimus dorsi (lats) muscle and helps you develop a more V shaped back..

Medium Grip is the one in which the space between your hands is equal to the width of your
shoulders.

Close Grip or the narrow angle grip is the one in which the distance between your hands is less
than the width of your shoulders. The close grip is a bit easier because it places shoulders and
elbows in an advantageous position and biceps pectoralis major also contribute.

*Target Muscle: Latissimus Dorsi (Lats), Biceps, Pectoralis Major*
*Type: Compound Back Exercise*

- Hold the pull up bar with your palms facing forwards.
- While holding the bar, extend both your arms and create a curvature on your lower back by bringing your torso back. This will be your starting position.
- Now exhale and gently pull your body upwards until your chest touches the bar. Put more strain on your back muscles on this fully contracted position. Only move your arms while going up and down and keep your torso steady and immobile.
- After you reach the top position, stay there a second and then slowly lower your body down and reach the starting position.
- Repeat this until the set is complete.
- If you are a beginner and lack the required strength to this exercise then you can either use a chin up machine or a spotter to hold your legs.
- If you are an advanced builder you can also do Weighted pull ups in which you wear a belt with an additional weights to increase the force requirements.

## 2. Lat Pull Downs

The equipment for exercise is pull down machine, in which a wide bar is attached to the pulley on top and linked to the weight.
*Target Muscle: Lats*
*Type: Compound Back Exercise*

- Sit on the machine and adjust the knee pad according to your height. These pads don't let your body to be lifted up by the weight.
- Hold the bar with your palms facing forwards. The grip can be varied according to your choice. In wide grip, your hands are spaced on the bar, wider than the width of your shoulders. In medium grip, they are spaced equal to the width of your

shoulder and in close grip; they are spaced at a distance lesser than the width of your shoulders.

- Hold the bars with both your arm in front of you and bring your torso back, forming a curvature on your lower back. Keep your chest out. This will be your starting position.
- Now gently pull the bar down while exhaling, until the bar touches your chest. Put more strain on your back in this position and keep your torso stationary and only move your arms.
- Keep in this position for a second and take a deep breath and raise the bar towards the starting position slowly.
- Repeat this cycle until the required repetitions are reached.

## 3. Rows with cable machine

You need a row machine with low pulley and V bar, for this exercise. You can also perform this exercise with barbell. This exercise is for your middle back.

*Target Muscles: Middle Back, Erecter Spinae and Paravertebral Muscles*
*Type: Compound Back Exercise*

- After sitting down on the machine. Put your feet on the platform with your knees slightly bent. This will be your starting position.
- Keeping the natural alignment of your back, lean forwards and hold the V bar handles.
- Now pull back the V bar and keep your arms fully extended. Your torso should be at 90 degrees with your leg. Keep your chest out and keep your back slightly arched. Hold the bar in front of you. This should be your starting position.
- Now pull the handle back towards your body until it touches your belly. Only move your arms and keep your core body stationary. Strain your middle back while breathing out.
- Stay in this contraction phase for a second and then gently go back to the

starting position as you inhale.

- Repeat the cycle until the desired number of repetitions is reached.
- Don't swing your back along with the movement as it can cause injury to your lower back.

## 4. Dumbbell Shrugs

Shrugs can be done with dumbbells, barbell and bands. The dumbbell shrugs are the most easy and effective. Shrugs target your upper back muscles.

*Target Muscles:   Trapezius*

*Type: Isolation Back Exercise*

- Hold the dumbbell in each hand and stand straight, keeping your arms on the side. Your palms should be facing your torso.
- Exhale and raise the dumbbells by lifting your shoulders as high as you can go. Stay in that position for a second.
- Go back to the starting position by lowering the dumbbells.
- Repeat the cycle until you reach the desired number of repetitions.
- Note that you should keep your arms extended all the time and do not flex the biceps at any time. Only move your shoulders.

## 5. Dead lifts

This exercise can be done with barbell, dumbbell, cable, band, axel and a lot of other things. The best type in gym settings is barbell dead lifts. This is the best exercise for your lower back.

This exercise should not be taken lightly, especially if you have a back problem. In that case, you should try the alternative in the form of cable Rows.

Do not use too much weight and do not round your back because this can cause injury to the back.

*Target Muscle: Hamstrings, Gluts, Lower Back, Psoas Major,*
*Type: Compound Exercise*

- Load the barbell and stand in front of it. Now keep your back straight and hold the bar at medium or shoulder width grip while bending your knees. That is your starting position. You can change your grip if you don't like it or you can also use wrist strap.
- Now, exhale and raise the bar by pushing the ground with your legs and also raising your upper body towards the erect position. When you reach the erect upright position, keep your chest out and contract your back. Keep your back straight at all the time
- Now bend your knees and lean your upper body forwards and put the bar slowly on the floor going back to the starting position. Keep your back straight throughout the cycle.
- Repeat the cycle until you reach your desired repetitions.

# Chest

## 1. Chest Dips

If you are a beginner and lack the strength to do this then you can use a dip assist machine which can assist you in pushing your body upwards. Or you can also use a spotter.
On the other hand, if you are an advanced builder, you can use weight belt to increase the resistance.

*Target Muscle: Chest, Pectoralis Major, Triceps*
*Type: Compound Chest Exercise*

- Stand between the two parallel bars of the chest dip machine and raise your body above the bars at arm's length. This is your starting position.
- Now, inhale and lower your body slowly while your elbows are flared outwards. You will feel a stretch in your chest.
- Now use the strength of your chest to raise your body back towards the starting position while exhaling. Make sure to contract your chest muscles on the top.
- Repeat the cycle until you reach the required number of repetitions.

## 2. Bench Press

This is one of the most effective and most popular exercises for the chest. It can be done by both dumbbells and barbell. It is also effective for your shoulders.

*Target Muscles: Chest, Pectoralis Major, Deltoid, Triceps.*
*Type: Compound Chest Exercise*

It can be done with different angles of the bench including flat, incline and decline. Changing the angle works the chest muscles in a different way. Incline bench presses put a greater emphasis onto the upper part of the pectoralis major muscle in the chest and shoulders while decline bench presses target the lower aspect. The flat bench press works the middle part of pectoralis major and deltoids. It is the best angle if you want strength.

**Barbell Bench Press:** Three grips can be used including wide, medium and narrow grip. Each grip burdens certain muscle groups. Narrow grip emphasizes more on your triceps. Medium grip is used more commonly. In this grip, the distance between your hands should be equal to the width of your shoulder. Medium grip creates an angle of 90 degrees between your arm and forearm in the middle of cycle. Wide grip emphasizes more on the shoulders along with chest muscles.

*CAUTION*: Perform this exercise very carefully and always keep a spotter with you. If a spotter is not available then lift lighter weights. Be in control of the barbell throughout the cycle.

- Hold the bar from the rack and keep it straight over your chest. Keep your arms locked. This is your starting position.
- Now, inhale and carefully lower the bar slowly until it touches your chest.
- After a second, exhale and push the bar back and slowly reach the starting position. Make sure to contract your chest muscle during this phase. Stay on the top for a second while keeping your arms locked. Now start coming down very slowly.
- Repeat this motion until you reach your desired number of reps
- Put the bar carefully back in the rack when you are done.

**Dumbbell Bench Press:** This exercise works on the same principle as the barbell bench press. Two dumbbells of appropriate weight are used.

- Hold a dumbbell in each hand and sit on a flat bench. Your palms should be facing each other. Hold the dumbbells up one by one and place them on your thighs.
- Now, lie down and keep the dumbbells at your shoulder width (medium grip). Now, rotate your wrists such that your palms are facing towards your knees. At this point there should be an angle of 90 degrees between your arm and forearm. That is your starting position.
- Now, exhale and push both the dumbbells upwards using your chest muscles. When you reach the top, lock your arms and stay that way for a second.
- Now slowly lower the dumbbells towards the starting position.
- Repeat this cycle until you reach the planned number of repetitions.
- Make sure that you are in control of dumbbells throughout the cycle. Put the dumbbells back on the floor carefully when you are done.

## 3. Pull over's (Straight Arm Dumbbell)

This exercise should be performed with extra caution and if you are a beginner then you should have a spotter to hand you over the dumbbell. Make sure that you hold the dumbbell carefully and it should not fall on you.

*Target muscles: Pectoralis Major (Chest)*
*Type: Isolation Chest Exercise*

- Put the dumbbell perpendicularly on a flat bench. Now lie on the bench perpendicularly, with only your shoulders touching the bench. Your body should make a cross with the bench. Your feet should be placed firmly on the floor and your hips should be below the level of the bench.
- Now hold the dumbbell with both hands. Raise the dumbbell and keep it at an arm's length above your chest. This is your starting position.
- Now, inhale and lower the dumbbell behind your head slowly in an arc. Go until you can feel a stretch on your chest muscles.

- Now exhale and bring the dumbbell back towards the starting position in the same arc. Stay in this position for a while.
- Repeat the cycle until you reach your desired number of repetitions.

## 4. Dumbbell Flyes

Flyes can be done with dumbbells and cable but as the dumbbells are easily available and effective, they are mentioned. You should be very careful during this exercise, like in any other exercise in which you need to lie down with the weight. Make sure that the dumbbells are new, intact and reliable.

*Target Muscle: Pectoralis Major (Chest)*
*Type: Isolation Chest Exercise*

- Take a dumbbell in each of your hands and lie down on the bench. Place the dumbbells on your thighs. You palms should be facing each other.
- Now, raise the dumbbells in front of you at shoulder width with the help of your thighs and lock your arms. This will be your starting point.
- Now, inhale and lower your arms on both sides in the form of an arc. Do this move with a slight flexion/bend on your elbow joint to prevent excessive load on your biceps. You will feel a stretch ay your chest muscles. Movement should only occur at your shoulder joints and your arms should be stationary throughout the cycle.
- Now exhale and return back up towards your starting position following the same arc. Stay in this position for one second.
- Repeat this until you reach your recommended number of repetitions.

# Shoulders

## 1. Military Press

It is a comprehensive and most effective exercise for shoulders (deltoids). It can be done with barbell, dumbbells and machine.

*Target Muscle: Deltoids (shoulders)*
*Type: Compound Shoulder Exercise*

**Barbell Military Press:** It is best if you do this exercise with a spotter to hand you the barbell especially if you are a beginner. Otherwise pick up the bar yourself carefully. The bar can be moved both behind and in front of the head. In my recommendation, front of the head is the safer option.

Your elbows can be either by your side or on your front during the motion. You can choose the way, which you find easy. I like to keep my elbows by my side because it covers a greater part of the deltoid muscle.

- Place a bar on a rack behind your head and sit on the military press bench. While holding the bar, your palms should be facing forwards. The recommended grip for this exercise is the wide grip, in which the distance between your hands is more than the width of your shoulder. This grip makes an angle of 90 degrees between your arm and forearm while going down during the motion.
- Now raise the bar above your head and lock your arms. The bar should be at a level, slightly in front of your head. This will be your starting position.
- Now, inhale and lower the bar to your collarbone.
-  Now exhale and lift the bar back to the starting position.
- Repeat this cycle until you reach the desired number of repetitions.
- The bar can also be placed behind the neck. But this variety is not recommended to the people with weak shoulders as it has a greater chance of injury to the rotator cuff because it can cause hyperextension of the shoulder joint by the weight of the barbell.

# Triceps

## 1. French Press

This exercise is best performed with barbell but it can also be performed with dumbbells, cables or a triceps blaster bar.

*Target Muscle:  Triceps Brachii*
*Type: Isolation Triceps Exercise*

- Hold a barbell and stand up with your palms facing forwards. This exercise is best done with a Close grip. (The distance between your hands should be less than your shoulder width.
- Now, raise the bar above your head by fully extending your arm. Do not bend your elbows. Your palms should be facing forwards. This is your starting position.
- Now, slowly lower the bar behind your head, in the form of an arc, until your forearm is perpendicular to the floor and it touches your biceps. Inhale, while doing this step.
- Now, exhale and raise the bar back towards the starting position. This step will cause the contraction in your triceps.
- Repeat the cycle until you reach the desired number of repetitions.

## 2. Tricep Extensions with Rope

You need a cable machine for this exercise. Select the weight and attach the rope with the pulley. Facing away from the machine, hold the rope with both hands.

*Target Muscle: Triceps Brachii*
*Type: Isolation Triceps Exercise*

- Your hands should go behind your head while holding the rope and your elbows should point straight up. Take a good stance by stabilizing your feet. Now, gently lean away from the machine to create more traction and stability. This is your starting position.

- Now, keeping your arm stationary, extend your elbow. Your arms will be raised above your head.
- Now slowly go back down and lower the weight, going back to the starting position.
- Repeat this cycle, until you reach the desired number of repetitions.

## 3. Tricep Dips

You need two parallel bars for dips. If you are a beginner and lack the strength to perform this exercise then you can use a spotter to help you raise your body. Or you can also use a dip assist exercise. On the other hand, if you are an advanced builder then you can use a weight belt to increase the amount of resistance.

*Target Muscle: Triceps*

*Type: Isolation Triceps Exercise*

- Raise your body with your arms, at an arm's length above the bars. Lock your arms at the top. This is your starting position.
- Now, slowly lower your body while inhaling. Keep your elbows close to your body and keep your torso straight and upright. Lower your body until the angle between your arms and forearms becomes 90 degrees.
- Now raise your body back up towards the starting position while exhaling. This movement will use your triceps.
- Repeat this cycle until the desired number of repetitions is reached.

# Biceps

## 2. Bicep Curls with Rotation

This exercise can be done in many ways. It can be done while sitting or standing. Either both arms can be used simultaneously or it can be performed by alternating arms.

*Target Muscle:  Biceps Brachii*
*Type: Isolation Biceps Exercise*

- Hold a dumbbell in both your hands and keep your elbows close to your body. Your palms should be facing your body at the starting position.
- Now, exhale and curl the weights using the biceps while keeping your upper arms stationary. Keep raising the dumbbells until they reach the shoulder level and your biceps are fully contracted. Stay in that position for a second or two.
- Now, lower the dumbbells slowly going back towards the starting position. Inhale while doing this step.
- Repeat the cycle until the desired number of repetitions is reached.

## 2. Bicep Curls with Barbell

This is a very good isolation exercise for Biceps. It only requires a barbell with a moderate weight. Alternatively, it can also be done with a straight bar, attached to a low pulley.

*Target muscle: Biceps Brachii*
*Type: Isolation bicep Exercise*

- Hold the barbell with a medium grip (shoulder width) while standing upright. Place your elbows close to our body. Your palms should be facing forward. This will be your starting position.
- Now exhale and start raising the bar contracting your biceps. Your arm should be stationary while this movement while only forearms should be moving.

- Raise the bar until it reaches the level of your shoulders and your biceps are fully contracted. Stay at that position for a second or two.
- Now, slowly lower the bar back towards the starting position as you inhale.
- Repeat the cycle until you reach the desired number of repetitions.

# Chapter 26

## <u>Scientific Laws of Building Muscle</u>

Ever wondered how a body responds to exercise the way it does? How can a thin lean man be converted into a big muscular man in just a few months? What are the processes going on inside the muscles?

All these questions will be answered in this section. I will try to give you an idea of the processes going on inside the muscle and its cells which lead to hypertrophy of that particular muscle.

### Adaptation Process

In order to get an understanding of the reason of the 'increased muscle mass in response to workout', we first have to learn about the process of adaptation.

I will also try to explain that why some people get different results than the others.

> <u>What Is Adaptation:</u> Adaptation is physiological process in which a person's body accustoms or adjusts itself to physical stress. In general, a limited amount of stress is good for you. It prepares you for handling further stress. That "preparation" is also known as adaptation. Something is true for the body building. When you put a certain amount of stress on a muscle regularly like lifting heavy weights, this muscle gradually prepares itself for lifting that kind of weight in the future.
>
> This is a natural physiological process and nature has made us that way.

> There is an order of these physiological changes that is followed to get the desired shape of the body. Giving stress to the body, which causes the body to adapt, which then changes its composition. So, the following three events should happen in order to bring about a change in body.
>
> 1. Stimulation by regular *stress* (Exercise)
> 2. Body *adapts* (in response to stress)
> 3. Body's composition is changed (*hypertrophy*)

> Note that I used the word regular above. I cannot emphasize that enough. ***Being regular is the key here.*** If you are not regular then your muscles do not get regular

stress and the adaptation process halts. So, hit the gym daily guys or that adaptation is not happening on its own!

## Muscular Hypertrophy and Microtrauma

➢ ***Muscular hypertrophy***: refers to the increase in the size of muscle cells which leads to an increase in an overall size of that muscle. Note that it does not mean an increase in "number" of muscle cells. This is the key process that is going on inside the muscles during bodybuilding.

The science behind the hypertrophy is the same as in adaptation. In fact, hypertrophy can be referred to as a "*result of adaptation process*".

Stress on a muscle stimulates adaptation and what is adaptation for muscle cells? It's Hypertrophy. If we put continuous progressive overload on the muscle cells (stress), they increase their size to tackle that stress. They store more nutrients in them and increase their protein synthesis. Eventually, they grow in size. This growth in the muscle cell size causes an overall increase in the muscle size and strength. This overall increase in size is termed as hypertrophy.(hyper- means more). Hence the hypertrophy can be achieved by strength training and anaerobic exercises. It can also be affected by a person's nutrition and certain drugs.

➢ **Microtrauma:** refers to the small damage to the muscle fibers that plays a very important role in growth of the muscle. These damaged muscle cells are replaced by addition of more (newer) muscle cells. This constant damage and regeneration causes a gradual increase in the muscle size.

The rule of nature is that, whenever any tissue of the body is injured, the body's response is to replace that damaged tissue. But when this damage (stress) is gradually increasing, then the body **overcompensates** by adding more tissue to that part. This happens due to increased growth rate and cell cycle in that tissue.

The same is true for muscle cells, when continuous and progressive stress is implied on the muscles, some of the muscle cells are damaged (microtrauma), the body adapts by regenerating the muscle cells and overcompensates by increasing cell cycle response. As a result the muscular size is increased along with the strength.

Hence all these terms are interlinked and are essential to understand the scientific and biological events in bodybuilding.

*Progressive overload causes stress, which cause microtrauma, which results in adaptation in the form of hypertrophy.*

# Progressive overload

Progressive overload is defined as the gradual increase in the stress applied to the body in strength training exercises. This process is applied in almost every form of strength training program including high intensity interval training, weight lifting and fitness training.

➢ The scientific programs involved in the progressive training include the adaptation process and hypertrophy. So, the same sequence of events happens in progressive overload. The stress causes the adaptation process, which causes the change in composition of body. But the difference is that the stress is **gradually increasing**. The muscles of the body are stressed in such a way that it starts the body's adaptive response even faster. Hence if you increase the weights or number of Reps gradually, your muscles will grow faster because of progressive overload.

➢ The stimulation of muscle hypertrophy is a single positive effect of progressive overload. It has a number of other advantages. Most important of which is its role in the development of stronger and denser bones. Not only bones but other connective tissues including tendons, ligaments and cartilage can also be positively affected by it. The body's blood flow to the exercising regions can be enhanced. When a muscle increases in size, its blood supply increases which ultimately increases the nerve connection between muscle and the brain.

- **Some ways to create progressive overload**

Here are some ways to increase the load on your muscles progressively, to achieve maximum muscular hypertrophy.

➢ Increase sets

- ➢ Increase resistance
- ➢ Increase intensity
- ➢ Increase frequency
- ➢ Increase exercises
- ➢ Decrease rest time
- ➢ Increase repetitions

**An example of progressive overload:**

Suppose that you perform Biceps Curl Barbell at 1×8 with 30 pounds. After some time your biceps grow in strength and size and then this exercise feels easier. After that period, your bicep will stop increasing in size and will maintain a plateau. This is due to lack of progressive overload. That is, your biceps adapted to a level which is required to do this particular exercise and there is no need for your bicep to increase further. If you create a progressive overload then there will be a need for them to grow bigger.

# Rate of Perceived Exertion (RPE)

| RPE Chart | |
|---|---|
| **Rate Of Perceived Exertion** | |
| 1 | Very Light Activity |
| 2-3 | Light Activity |
| 4-6 | Moderate Activity |
| 7-8 | Vigorous Activity |
| 9 | **Very Hard Activity** |
| 10 | **Max. Effort Activity** |

➢ Rate of Perceived Exertion or RPE is a method to measure the intensity of an exercise. It is usually used in research settings, but it can also be used in assessing the intensity of a training program.

➢ This is a subjective scale and is based on how hard your body perceives/feels the workout.
It is also called Borg CR10 scale. It ranges from 1 to 10 in increasing perception of work, 1 being very light activity and 10 being maximum effort activity.

➢ It is based on how you feel after doing an exercise and how your body perceives that exercise.
In the normal settings, you should at least exercise at 4 or 5 level.

➢ Make sure to include your stress and tiredness level in determining your RPE. It is just to get a rough idea about the intensity of an exercise.

# Range of Motion (ROM)

➢ Range of motion or ROM is defined as the distance, a joint can move between its completely flexed and completely extended position in a particular direction. This term is frequently used in weightlifting and medical communities. Every particular joint has a specific range of motion. ROM can be decreased due to certain injuries and then certain exercises can be done to increase it to a normal level.

➢ The reason for mentioning ROM here is that during exercise, you should perform an effective full range of motion. Some people like to do partial range of motion but it may predispose your muscles and tendons to injuries.In order to get maximum results you should do full effective range of motion.

# Time under Tension (TUT)

➢ The time under tension or TUT is defined as the time during which, a muscle is under stress in an exercise. It is used to determine the duration of stress in a particular exercise, as it is a key factor for muscle growth. The longer you keep a muscle under stress, the more it will grow. Because more stress will cause more micro trauma, more adaptation and more hypertrophy.

➢ An average set of 10 reps takes about 15-20 seconds. For an optimum muscle growth, you should time your set, such that it lasts around 30 to 40 seconds.

Now the question is how to increase time under tension. Here are some easy ways:

- Keep a steady tempo of your exercise.
- Keep a watch or timer with you, always.
- Don't spend a lot of time at the easy portion of the exercise (e.g. at the top in Military press)
- Don't compromise form to adjust the time.
- Spend more time in the toughest portion of the exercise

# Chapter 27

## **Plan Everything; Set Goals**

A person's life is like a journey. Aim is the destination towards which he is moving. Once he reaches that destination, he decides to reach another destination and sets out in that direction. Can one imagine what would the life be like if there is no direction? The person would be like a lost passenger who is just travelling unknown of the direction in which he is moving and that makes no sense.

Body building or workout also has a same rule. There should be a particular plan and goals should be set in order to achieve something. Otherwise it becomes illogical as a passenger unknown of his destination.

### Aim

Aim is a long term plan which a person makes at any step and strives towards it with full force. It is very important in body building to make an aim which a person needs to achieve. Aim could be like how much weight a person wants to lose in one year or what kind of shape he wants for his body to achieve for which he is going through the effort.

Every person has different priority and they choose their aim according to it. Some are doing it for a better shape of body, some want their bodies to be superior to others while some start body building to attract other people. One thing should be kept in mind that aims regarding body building should be moderate and according to capability. If we make heroic aims, it becomes difficult and we often find ourselves dispersed from the main course. After achieving that aim, the person chooses other destination and starts off to achieve it.

### Goals

When a passenger has a long distance to travel, he makes small milestones in his mind like where to make stops and how much time needed to travel that long. Goals are like that. These are the milestones a person chooses in pursuit of the aim.

In body building, setting goals is very important for two main reasons. One reason is that it is almost impossible to go the whole distance without making a stop and reviewing the achievements so one needs to make small halts. The other main reason is that it gives lots of confidence and encouragement when a person reaches a milestone in a particular time frame. He believes in himself that he is capable of achieving anything if he wants to achieve.

## Goals in Body Building

When you set a goal for yourself, don't go to either extreme. No one can get all shredded in a week. Take a moderate approach instead. Following points should be kept in mind while making goals

- They should be according to the priorities.
- There should always be a variety so that a person does not wear off his routine.
- Don't be over ambitious as it will lead to non-compliance.
- Set a role model or an inspiration will be quite helpful.
- Remember that it will take time to achieve desired results.
- Consistency is the key to a good shaped body and should always be consistence.

# Chapter 28

## Why Cheat Days are Bad?

Like a relationship, bodybuilding or workout depends on the fact that the person remains loyal and does not cheat. If one cheats in a relationship, he/she has to suffer consequences or maybe a breakup. Cheating in bodybuilding is not as severe as cheating in a relationship but still results in loss of quite a workup which a person has to now start again.

### What are Cheat days?

As already mentioned that body building is not only dependent on exercise but it also requires modification in life style, especially diet has to be changed to get much better results. A person who wishes to gain an ideal weight or an ideal physique should have a good control on his diet.

Cheat days, rather over eating days, are some days on which a body builder forgets all his diet plans and eats as much and whatever he wants. Some people consider as a reward after continuous days of strenuous exercise and withdrawal from tasty food.

### What happens on cheat days?

During body building, a person withdraws from all the tasty, rather fattening, pleasures of the world. On a particular cheat days, he forgets all his diet plans and eat throughout the day those things which some time ago were responsible for his uneven body shape. The main charms of those days include burgers, fried chicken, bacon, fried products, cakes, sweet things, fast food of different types and all those things which were prohibited during workout schedule.

### Cheat days are bad

Some trainers consider cheat days as a reward or positive reinforcement after a trainee reaches a particular goal. They think that it causes an increase in the morale of the person and the trainee feels more encouraged but what they don't consider that it has the ability to stray the person from the modified life style which is necessary for workout.

When a person celebrates cheat days it can cause many harms, first of which is the regain of all that weight which took so many days to burn. The person realizes all the tastes which he had to withdraw and may leave workout for the better of his tongue. Some of the times, the person thinks that it is okay to eat unhealthy for some time considering the fact that if he is allowed a complete day to cheat, there would be less harm if he eats some every day or after some days.

## Cheat days are not recommended

"No pain, no gain". This saying is so true regarding body building that it seems it was made for this particular context. There is no easy path and no shortcut. If a person wants to lose some weight, acquire ideal figure, or a model like body which attracts everyone, he has to remember that he has to leave the pleasures of tongue and focus on much bigger aim which is to acquire a perfect shape. It might seem tough at the beginning, but once a person starts seeing changes, he feels confident and knows that he can live without cheating his body. So, it is recommended that one should be loyal with his aim in order to be successfully able to achieve it.

# Chapter 29

## <u>Some Simple Ways to Eliminate Cravings</u>

Man is a social animal. The addition of being social does not disprove that he does not have animal instincts. These instincts include cravings. Cravings can be of different types. Some have cravings for more and more money; others have cravings for power while some have sexual cravings (about which I am not going to talk about much to the disappointment of readers). The craving harmful to the body building is for food and must be controlled and eliminated.

Food is a necessity of life but for some people it becomes opposite and life becomes necessary for eating food. Such people can be seen as having a round abdomen and uneven body. The craving for food is a major threat in such a person when he decides to change the way he looks to a more pleasing appearance.

**How Cravings Start**

Craving for food can occur at any time to any person either he works out or not because let's face it, everyone likes to eat yummy food. It is also a known fact that yummier the food, more it affects shape of the body. If a person is eating a nice juicy burger or a sweet and lovely looking piece of cake near you, how can you not be tempted to have some of it? Major problem occurs due to the friends who are not working or are not concerned about their body shape. They tend to eat such food that is tasty but unhealthy for a person who works out and it becomes difficult to follow the diet plan.

Fast food chains are the other major enemy of the body. They post such tempting ads and people talk about their variety of tasty food, it almost becomes like a person is torturing by not eating that tasty food.

**Controlling Cravings**

It is one of the most difficult parts of the body building procedure and requires lots of self-control and a very strong will power. It takes a man with a determined man to face his cravings and then control himself leading to elimination of such interests. Some of the points which can help in this manner are as follows

- **Look in the mirror:** This is a very easy method to control the cravings. When a person is tempted to eat some non-healthy food, just look at the mirror with shirt on or off. If a person has round abdomen and visible fat, it will decrease his appetite and if he has nice shaped abs, it will make him feel that such food can destroy it.
- **Avoid eating in company:** as it will make it much difficult to control temptations if someone is eating a juicy burger in front.
- **Eat a variety of food:** the food which a person eats should be varied so that the person does not become bored of same type of food and be tempted to cheat on his diet.
- **Stay busy:** because when a person has lot of free time and has nothing to do, he will eat more and more to pass the time.
- **Eat after short intervals:** so that the person is never hungry and does not have physiological craving to eat.

# Chapter 30

# The No-BS Guide To Supplements

Supplements are additions people take to increase their performance and body shape. Note that many products out there are pure BS and you should rather focus on a good diet. Supplements will never be better than real food!

## List of Supplements

Some of the useful supplements which are generally used are as follows

### CREATINE MONOHYDRATE:

Our muscles normally contain creatine phosphate in stored form and it is the energy source which enables our muscles to keep contracting. Creatine is usually used with flavored powders and mixed with liquid. It enhances the body's ability to produce energy rapidly. With more energy, you can train harder and more often, producing faster results.  Research shows that creatine is most effective in high-intensity training and explosive activities. It is also an osmotically active agent which brings water into muscle cells and increase protein synthesis. When this stored form is empty, it is very difficult to continue work out. Creatine, if taken before workout can enable one to use muscles for a longer period of time with lots of energy.

*How to take it:* Start with 20 grams loading dose for 5-7 days. After 5-7 days, maintenance dose of 5 grams per day should be taken for rest of the cycle

You can also take a more customized approach based on your body mass. According to this formula take 0.3 grams per Kg of the body weight for first 5-7 days. The maintenance dose of 0.03 gram per kg is taken for the rest of the cycle. The ideal use is before  and after your workout. An optimal cycle would be taking Creatin for 8 weeks, then taking 2 weeks off.

### GLUTAMINE:

It is a naturally found and most abundant amino acid present in the body which we get from the diet and helps in dealing with all daily stress one experiences in everyday life . Glutamine plays key roles in protein metabolism, anti-catabolism and cell volumizing. Glutamine also increases the ability to secrete Human Growth Hormone, which helps metabolize body fat and support new muscle growth. Glutamine's anti-catabolism ability prevents the breakdown of muscles. One of its advantages which makes it a perfect supplement is that it has no side effect at all. Pre workout intake can enhance timing of workout.

*How to take it:* 20-40 grams per day is enough during workout days. While on off days, 10 grams per day is sufficient. The Ideal time to use it is before workout.

## ARGININE

L-Arginine has an amazing nitrogen retension ability and is therefore added to many supplements. As we all know, nitrogen is the most important element in the muscle protein synthesis.

It enhances our immune system by increasing the activity of thymus gland and hence increases the production of T cells. Arginine has the ability to to stimulate the release of insulin from pancreas and Growth hormone from the pituitary. Both these hormones help in gaining muscle mass. Arginine is also known for improving the health of liver, skin and connective tissue and it also increases the  sexual stimulus.
Naturally, it is present in whole wheat, soy, rice, raisins and seeds.

*How to take it:* There is no recommended dosage for this amino acid because it is mostly mixed with other supplements and proein shakes. Free form arginine is rarely manufactured. But if you have to choose between two equal products, select the one containing more arginine.

## PROTEIN SHAKES

A convenient method of having protein is in the form of protein powder mixed with soy milk or water. Most commonly used plant based substances include soy powder,  pea proteins, rice proteins etc. Regardless of the good protein shakes do for our bodies, they can sometimes be a little hard to swallow because of their bland taste. One can add some flavor to the shakes which may be in the form of vanilla, strawberry, oatmeal, cocoa powder and different dry fruits like almond, pistachio etc. For each recipe, put all the ingredients into a blender and blend until the shake reaches the desired consistency. Depending on your macronutrient and caloric needs and taste preferences, one may need to alter the recipes. Don't be afraid to improvise!  Post workout intake is beneficial.

*How to take it:* 40 grams per day intake is more than enough in those intending to build body. Pre and post workout are the best times for intake.

## BRANCHED CHAIN AMINO ACIDS:

These make about 33% of total protein content of body. These include leucine, anti-leucine and valine. These amino acids work together to prevent muscle breakdown. Branched chain amino acid supplementation is very useful for gaining mass, but their main work lies in maintaining muscle mass while on a calorie-deficit diet.

They're particularly useful for bodybuilding competitors who take their physiques to the lean extreme. During these extremes, body may face catabolic crisis in which its major compounds like proteins may start breaking down to generate energy. These amino acids are helpful in saving the main essence of muscles i.e proteins.

*How to take it:* 3:1:1 ratio of leucine to isoleucine to valine. 5 grams to 10 grams both before and after workouts is an ideal dose.

## FATTY ACIDS:

These can be obtained from chia seeds, flax seed oil, many nuts and are very important part of muscle building. Fats help to provide lots of energy for the workout and also help in maintaining the nervous system and level of different hormones in the body.

*How to take it:* Approximately 1 tablespoon per 100 pounds of body weight is useful.

## RHODIOLA ROSEA:

A research has shown that those who took Rhodiola Rosea before and after workout have shown better results and increased endurance capacity. Rhodiola rosea can boost energy and treat mental fatigue, along with other conditions. Rhodiola rosea relieves stress by balancing the body's stress-response system. With constant stress, a person feels edgy, tired, or depressed. Rhodiola rosea helps re-establish balance by strengthening the body's response to physical, mental, and emotional stressors.

*How to take it:* It is most commonly found in a standardized extract that contains rosavins and salidrosides in a 3:1 ratio.

## CALCIUM:

Calcium is very important in performing lots of functions in the body and also a very important component of muscle contraction. The level of calcium in the body is naturally maintained by hormones which control its level in blood and on the bones. It has a key role in osmoregulation and involved in several functions like clotting, strengthening of bones and teeth. Its major role in body building is that it allows muscle contraction. In the absence of it or decreased amount muscles cannot release them from a tight state. It can be obtained from vegetables like kale and bok choy which have large amounts of calcium.

## IRON:

Iron is a major component of our body's functioning. It is the central atom of hemoglobin which is present in red blood cells and is responsible for transportation of oxygen in all parts of body. It is also central atom of a protein called myoglobin present in muscles which permits storage of oxygen and results in more energy production for muscles contraction.It's several other functions include being part of many enzymes and hence control major reactions in the body. It can be obtained from fruits like apple, leafy green vegetables such as spinach, Swiss chard, broccoli rabe, bok choy, and asparagus.

## FLAX SEED OIL:

It is a very good source of omega 3 fatty acids which are considered good for the body's

*How to take it:* Approximately 1 tablespoon per 100 pounds of body weight per day.

## BETAINE:

It is a muscle-building compound naturally present in whole grains and spinach. It is helpful in gaining muscle strength and decreases body fat percentage. Betaine works by increasing protein synthesis in the body, which helps build muscle after tough workouts.

*How to take it:* 1.25 grams twice a day is ideal dose.

## BETA ALANINE:

During strong exercise, lactic acid accumulates in the muscles resulting in fatigue and burning sensation in the muscles. When there is extra beta-alanine, muscles can work longer and harder without the acid buildup as it acts as an acid buffer.
*How to take it:* A dose of 1.2 grams per day is most effective. Pre workout intake is beneficial.

## CAFFEINE:

Caffeine is an effective sports supplements easily available kitchen cabinet. It helps improve performance and power output, decreases symptoms of fatigue, helps to work longer and stronger, and acts as a mental focusing agent. It is also regarded as a fat burner since it melts down fat in the body.

*How to take it:* It is easily available in the form of coffee. Caffeine pills are also present but it is important to control the amount of the drug. Start with a low dose of 50 milligrams, and increase up to 300 milligrams.

www.ingramcontent.com/pod-product-compliance
Lightning Source LLC
Chambersburg PA
CBHW050456290526
45786CB00006B/2312